Communication Skills in Pharmacy Practice

A Practical Guide for Students and Practitioners

FOURTH EDITION

Communication Skills in Pharmacy Practice

A Practical Guide for Students and Practitioners

FOURTH EDITION

William Tindall, Ph.D., R.Ph.
Professor
Department of Family Medicine
School of Medicine
Wright State University
Dayton, Ohio

Robert S. Beardsley, Ph.D., R.Ph.
Professor and Associate Dean
School of Pharmacy
University of Maryland
Baltimore, Maryland

Carole L. Kimberlin, Ph.D.
Professor
Pharmacy Health Care Administration
College of Pharmacy
University of Florida

LIPPINCOTT WILLIAMS & WILKINS
A **Wolters Kluwer** Company

Philadelphia • Baltimore • New York • London
Buenos Aires • Hong Kong • Sydney • Tokyo

Editor: David Troy
Managing Editor: Matthew J. Hauber
Marketing Manager: Paul Jarecha
Production Editor: Paula C. Williams
Designer: Armen Kojoyian
Compositor: Inhouse Composition
Printer: RR Donnelley & Sons - Crawfordsville

Library of Congress Cataloging-in-Publication Data

Communication skills in pharmacy practice : a practical guide for students and practitioners / [edited by] William Tindall, Robert S. Beardsley, Carole L. Kimberlin.— 4th ed.
    p.cm.
Includes bibliographical references and index.
ISBN 0-7817-3295-6
   1. Communication in pharamcy. 2. Pharmacist and patietn. I. Tindall, William N. II. Beardsley, Robert S. III. Kimberlin, Carole L.

RS56 .C65 2002
615′.1′014—dc21

To Sylvia, Christine and Laura;
Kathy, Kyle;
and Philip
for
Communicating the Lessons of Love

CONTRIBUTORS
(Chapter 11)

Betsy L. Sleath, Ph.D.
Associate Professor of Pharmaceutical
   Policy and Evaluative Sciences
University of North Carolina School of Pharmacy

Patricia J. Bush, Ph.D.
Professor Emeritus
Georgetown University School of Medicine

Preface

This textbook has been created to help pharmacists be more effective educators and advocates for patients and more successful managers and employees. The first three editions of this textbook found wide acceptance in over 60 pharmacy colleges in the United States, Canada, United Kingdom, Australia, and other countries where pharmacy curricula are changing from a product-focused to a patient-centered orientation. Feedback from students, practitioners, professors, and others has indicated support for this fourth edition. We appreciate the helpful feedback from our readers and colleagues. In this fourth edition, readers will find new principles, practices, and procedures that contribute to the pharmacist's ability to promote good health outcomes for patients. We have crafted our revisions with continuing admiration for our profession and for those pharmacists who are working diligently to improve patient care.

This book rests on a foundation of three interlocking parts. Part I focuses on defining interpersonal communication and its various components. The purpose of this section is to help readers better understand communication, which can be a complex and fragile process, and to appreciate the importance of effective communication to their success as pharmacists. Part II describes practical skills for pharmacists. This section provides insights into the complexities of professional interaction along with a strong focus on the practical application of communication skills to pharmacy practice. The goal of Part III is to reveal how pharmacists can apply these skills to everyday encounters to promote patient care and meet the needs of others.

Unfortunately, some pharmacy practice environments are not conducive to productive interpersonal communication. In fact, some skeptics might urge that pharmacists should not be concerned with communication skill development, since pharmacists do not interact with patients very often. We recognize that interpersonal communication is limited in many practice environments because of certain work place factors. However, the fact that these situations exist should not prevent pharmacists from trying to improve interpersonal communication no matter how challenging the environment. We try to address many of these practice issues and provide strategies about how to enhance the interactions that do occur.

In summary, interpersonal communication often appears to be a simple process at first glance. However, as revealed in this book, interpersonal skill development is a complex process requiring a life-long commitment to improvement and practice. Pharmacists must acknowledge the value of interpersonal communication as the foundation of trust between patients and pharmacists. Pharmacists have a covenantal responsibility to not only dispense appropriate medications but also ensure patient understanding of what they are used for, what patients can expect from them, and what outcomes could be expected. We hope you enjoy the journey to learning more about this important process.

William N. Tindall
Dayton, Ohio

Robert S. Beardsley
Baltimore, Maryland

Carole L. Kimberlin
Gainesville, Florida

Contents

Chapter 1

Introduction: Patient-Centered Communication in Pharmacy Practice

▓ OVERVIEW

To meet their professional responsibilities, pharmacists have become more patient-centered in providing pharmaceutical care. Pharmacists have the potential to contribute even more powerfully to improved patient care through efforts to reduce medication errors and other causes of medication-related morbidity. Meeting this potential requires pharmacists to establish new relationships with patients—relationships that create true "partnerships" with patients in helping them reach their therapeutic goals.

INTRODUCTION

Pharmacists are accepting more responsibility in ensuring that patients reach desired outcomes with their medication therapy. This changing role requires pharmacists to switch from a medication-centered or task-centered practice to patient-centered care. Patient-centered care depends on the pharmacist's ability to develop trusting relationships with patients, to engage in an open exchange of information, to involve patients in the decision-making process regarding treatment, and to help them reach therapeutic goals that both the patients and their health care providers endorse. Effective communication is central to meeting these patient care responsibilities in the practice of pharmacy.

Pharmacist Responsibility in Patient Care

The cost to society associated with medication-related morbidity and mortality is of growing concern (Ernst and Grizzle, 2001; Hepler and Strand, 1990; Johnson and Bootman, 1995; Manasse, 1989). The Institute of Medicine report on patient safety concluded that medication-related errors are among the most prevalent errors in medical care (Committee on Quality of Health Care in America, 1999). The potential of pharmacists to play a pivotal role in reducing incidence of both medication-related errors and drug-related illness is also receiving increased attention (Hepler, 2001; Hepler and Strand, 1990; Leape et al, 1999).

Hepler and Strand (1990) have made a compelling case for the societal need for pharmaceutical care, which they define as "the responsible provision of drug therapy for the purpose of achieving definite outcomes that improve a patient's quality of life." Professional pharmacy associations have changed their mission statements in recent years to reflect the increased responsibility that pharmacists are being asked to assume for the appropriate use of drugs in society. Such an expanded role for pharmacists is also mandated under provisions of the Omnibus Budget Reconciliation Act of 1990 (OBRA 90).

Under provisions of the OBRA legislation, pharmacists were expected to obtain information from Medicaid patients or their caregivers as well as to provide information to patients for the purpose of preventing or identifying and resolving potential medication-related problems. Pharmacists must maintain patient profiles that contain patient demographic information, a comprehensive list of medications being taken, allergies, adverse drug reactions, disease states, and pharmacist comments relevant to an individual patient's drug therapy. This database can allow pharmacists to fulfill the OBRA requirement of prospective drug use review. Such a review involves examination of a patient's records before dispensing a medication in order to identify and resolve any potential problems. These problems may include overutilization, underutilization, therapeutic duplication, drug–drug interactions, incorrect drug dosage, drug allergy problems, incorrect duration of drug treatment, clinical abuse or misuse, and drug–disease contraindications. In addition, pharmacists are required to offer to engage in a discussion of a patient's therapy whenever a medication is dispensed. Under this provision, a pharmacist must offer to counsel patients on their medications (both new and refill) to prevent or identify/resolve problems with medication use.

The "patient-centered" role envisioned by pharmacy mission statements and OBRA 90 provisions would afford pharmacists a value to society far beyond that provided by their current "drug-centered" role. In fact, neither drug products nor dispensing tasks per se are essential to a patient-centered mission. They are simply *means* of achieving specified goals in individual patients. The goals are those *outcomes* of therapy that improve a patient's health and quality of life.

However, although the mission statements of professional organizations can help guide practice, they must be translated into patient care activities that pharmacists provide to each of their patients. The interpersonal relationships that professionals develop with patients require effective communication skills and are necessary in meeting a professional mission for pharmacy.

Importance of Communication in Meeting Patient Care Responsibilities

The communication process between health professionals and patients serves two primary functions:

1. It establishes the ongoing relationship between the provider and the patient.
2. It provides the exchange of information necessary to assess a patient's health condition, implement treatment of medical problems, and evaluate the effects of treatment on a patient's quality of life.

Establishing a trusting relationship with a patient is not something that is simply a "nice thing to do." The quality of the patient–provider relationship is crucial. All professional activities between a pharmacist and a patient take place in the context of the relationship they establish. An effective relationship forms the base that allows a pharmacist to meet professional responsibilities in patient care.

The purpose of the professional–patient relationship and of the activities engaged in must constantly be kept in mind. The essential goal is to be able to achieve mutually understood and agreed-upon health outcomes that improve a patient's quality of life. Pharmacist activities must therefore be thought of in terms of the patient outcomes that pharmacists help to reach. We must begin to redefine what we do with the focus being on patient need. Our goal, for example, is changed from providing patients with drug information to a goal of ensuring that patients understand their treatment and thus can take medications safely and appropriately. The pharmacist's goal is not to get patients to do as they are told (i.e., comply) but to help them reach intended treatment outcomes.

Providing information or trying to improve patient compliance must each be seen as a means of reaching a desired outcome rather than an end in itself. Even communication with a patient is not an end in itself. Conversation between patient and health professional has a purpose that is different from that of conversation between friends. Patient–professional communication is a means to an end—that of establishing a therapeutic relationship to effectively provide health care services that the patient needs. It is the patient's well-being that is paramount. Professionals, because of their unique knowledge and special societal responsibilities, must bear the greater burden in ensuring effective communication in patient–professional encounters.

What Is Patient-Centered Care?

Mead and Bower (2000) describe five dimensions of patient-centered medical care (summarized in Box 1.1):

1. Practitioners must understand the social and psychological as well as the biomedical factors that relate to the illness experience of a patient.
2. Providers must perceive the "patient as person." This requires understanding the patient's unique experience of illness and the "personal meaning" it entails.
3. Providers must share power and responsibility. The ideal relationship is more egalitarian than is traditionally seen, with patients more actively involved in dialogue and in the decision-making surrounding treatment.
4. Providers must promote a "therapeutic alliance." This involves incorporating patient perceptions of the acceptability of interventions; mutually agreed-upon goals for treatment; and a trusting, caring relationship between health professional and patient. The perception that a provider "cares" is essential to patient trust. Examination of reasons for filing malpractice claims against providers suggest that patient anger over a perceived lack of caring from providers and dissatisfaction with provider communication were important elements in decisions to file (Hickson et al, 1992).
5. Providers must be aware of their own responses to patients and the sometimes unintended effects their behaviors may have on patients.

Box 1.1 PROVIDING PATIENT-CENTERED CARE

The pharmacist must be able to:

- Understand the illness experience of the patient
- Perceive each patient's experience as unique
- Foster a more egalitarian relationship with patients
- Build a "therapeutic alliance" with patients to meet mutually understood goals of therapy
- Develop self-awareness of personal effects on patients

Understanding Medication Use from the Patient Perspective

Models of the prescribing process that are "practitioner-centered" have primarily focused on decisions made and actions taken by physicians and other health care providers. The patient is "acted upon" rather than being portrayed as an active participant who makes ongoing decisions affecting the outcomes of treatment. The patient is viewed as the object of professional ministrations and as the cooperative (or recalcitrant) follower of professional dictates.

One of our professional conceits is that writing the prescription and dispensing the drug are the key acts in the medication use process. However, in most cases, it is the patient or the patient's caregiver who must return home and carry out the prescribed treatment. Drug therapy is the most ubiquitous of medical interventions and, in ambulatory care, is largely managed by the patient. The degree of autonomy that is possible with medication therapy in noninstitutionalized patients makes it likely that patients will make decisions and assert control over treatment in various ways. Many patients make autonomous decisions to alter treatment regimens—decisions that may be made without consultation or communication with health care providers (Conrad, 1985; Donovan & Blake, 1992; Trostle, 1988). Ignorance of patient-initiated decisions on medication use, in turn, makes it difficult for health care professionals to accurately evaluate the effects of drug treatment.

Although providers no doubt view autonomous patient behavior as ill advised, it would be more helpful to acknowledge the fact that patients do exercise ultimate control over drug treatment. Rather than trying to stifle patient autonomy, it would be more productive for health professionals to strengthen the therapeutic alliance with patients by increasing the level of patient participation and control in decisions that are made about treatment.

Encouraging a More Active Patient Role in Therapeutic Monitoring

Providers, including pharmacists, could do more to enable patients and their family or caregivers to take a more active role in monitoring response to treatment and in informing providers about response to treatment. The information that a patient provides as part of therapeutic monitoring is essential to ensuring that therapeutic goals are being met. Although INR (international normalized ratio) or Hb A_{1c} (glycosylated hemoglobin) values may provide the comfort of a scientific basis for therapeutic monitoring, for many chronic conditions providers must rely, in whole or in part, on the patient's report of response to treatment. Treatment of depression and pain, for example, has the patient self-report as the only basis of evaluation of response to therapy. Many other conditions such as asthma, angina, gastroesophageal reflux disease, epilepsy, and arthritis rely heavily on the patient's report of symptoms.

In addition to conditions in which patient report of symptoms is critical to monitoring, research has documented the beneficial effects on patient outcomes of increased patient involvement in self-monitoring of physiological indicators of treatment effectiveness. Certainly, patient self-monitoring of blood glucose has become standard practice in managing diabetes. In addition, blood glucose awareness training programs (BGAT) teach patients to recognize signs of both hyperglycemia and hypoglycemia. The BGAT training programs have been found to improve a patient's ability to accurately estimate blood glucose fluctuations and prevent severe hypoglycemic episodes (Cox et al, 2001; Cox et al, 1994). Programs to increase patient participation in monitoring of coagulation therapy along with protocol-based patient management of warfarin dosing have led to reduced incidence of major bleeding in patient monitoring intervention groups (Beyth et al, 2000). These studies point to the sophistication with which patients can monitor their response to therapy and make informed decisions when they are taught how to interpret both symptomatic experience and results of physiological tests.

Other programs have designed interventions to teach patients how to be more assertive in obtaining information from providers. Intervention group subjects were found to be more likely than control subjects to question providers following the training intervention (Greenfield et al, 1985, 1988; Kaplan et al, 1989; Kimberlin et al, 2001; Roter, 1984). In addition, patient follow-up found that intervention group patients had improved health outcomes, including improved glycemic control in diabetic patients, for up to a year after the interventions (Greenfield et al, 1985; Kaplan et al, 1989).

The Joint Commission on Accreditation of Healthcare Organizations (JCAHO) and the Agency for Healthcare Research and Quality

(AHRQ) have published tips for patients to empower them to be more active in their own treatment and in decisions made on their care (AHRQ, 2000; JCAHO, 2002). As an example, one tip for surgery patients from JCAHO states: "Ask to have the surgical site marked with a permanent marker and to be involved in marking the site. This means that the site cannot be easily overlooked or confused (for example, surgery on the right knee instead of the left knee)." Another piece of advice states: "Make sure you get the results of all tests and procedures. Ask the doctor or nurse when and how you will get the results. Don't assume the results are ok if you don't get them when expected."

A Patient-Centered View of the Medication Use Process

A patient-centered view of the medication use process focuses on the patient's role in the process. The medication use process for noninstitutionalized patients begins when the patient perceives a health care need or health-related problem. This is experienced as a deviation from what is "normal" for the individual. It may be the experience of symptoms or other sort of lifestyle interruption that challenges or threatens the patient's sense of well-being. The patient then interprets the perceived problem. This interpretation is influenced by a host of psychological and social factors unique to the individual. These include the person's previous experience with the formal health care system; family influences; cultural differences in the conceptualization of "health" and "illness"; knowledge of the problem (individuals vary greatly in the level of medical and biological knowledge); health beliefs that may or may not coincide with accepted medical "truths"; psychological characteristics; personal values, motives, and goals; and so on. In addition, the patient's interpretation may be influenced by outside forces, such as family members who offer their own interpretations and advice.

The patient may take no action to treat, either because the problem is seen as minor or transitory or because the patient lacks the means to initiate treatment. If the patient takes action, the action can include initiation of self-treatment, initiation of contact with a nonmedical provider (e.g., a faith healer), or contact with a health care provider. If the patient takes action that involves contact with a health care professional, whether it is a physician, pharmacist, or other health care practitioner, he or she must describe the "symptom" experience and to some extent his or her interpretation of that experience. In many ways, it is at this point that control gets transferred from the patient to the professional, for it is the professional who can legitimize the experience by giving it a name (diagnosis). Such an act, however, transforms the experience from that with patient meaning into that with practitioner meaning (which may or may not be shared by the patient). The quality of the professional assessment depends, in part, on the thoroughness of the patient report, the skill of the practitioner in eliciting relevant information, and the receptivity of the professional to "hear" information that is potentially important. The practitioner's skill in communicating information about the diagnosis may alter or refine the patient's conceptualization of his or her illness experience, making patient understanding more congruent with that of the practitioner.

After the health care provider reaches a professional assessment or diagnosis of the patient's problem based on patient report, patient examination, and other data, he or she makes a recommendation to the patient. If the recommendation is to initiate drug treatment, the patient may or may not carry out the recommendation. The patient may have a variety of reasons for doing this, such as economic constraints, a lack of understanding of the purpose of the recommendation, or failure to "buy into" the treatment plan. Some of these patient decisions may reflect a failure in the communication process between provider and patient.

When patients do accept the recommendation to initiate drug treatment, obtain the medication, and attempt to follow the regimen as prescribed, they can do so only according to their ability to understand how the drugs are intended to be taken. For many patients, medication-taking may include misunderstanding of what is being recommended or unintended deviations from the prescribed treatment regimen (e.g., doses are forgotten). Alternatively, patients may administer the drug but intentionally modify the regimen. In both unintentional and intentional modifications of prescribed treatment, the patient's actions may be influenced by how well providers succeeded in establishing a mutually understood and agreed-upon treatment plan.

Regardless of the medication-taking practices that patients establish, they evaluate the consequences of the treatment in terms of perceived benefits and perceived costs or barriers. This evaluation results in patients (a) continuing with the drug treatment practices essentially as they have been established, (b) altering their drug treatment regimens, or (c) discontinuing drug treatment. In any case, patients are continuously estimating what they perceive the effects of their actions to be and adjusting their behavior accordingly. It is inevitable that, as patients begin drug treatment, they will monitor their own response. In other words, they will decide whether or not they feel differently, and they will look for signs that the treatment is effective or for indications that there may be a problem with the drug. The problem is not that patients monitor their response to medications—it is inevitable and desirable that they do so. The problem is that patients often lack information on what to expect from treatment; on what to look for that will give them valid feedback on their response to the medication. Lacking this information, they apply their own common-sense criteria.

Patients may interrupt the treatment process by failing to contact providers when follow-up is expected, which may involve discontinuing participation in the formal health care system for a period of time or contacting a new provider and beginning the whole process again. Of the patients who do contact the provider, some will communicate their perceptions, problems, and decisions regarding treatment. Other patients may contact providers and *not* convey this information (or not convey all pertinent aspects). This follow-up contact occurs during revisits with a physician or refills of prescriptions from pharmacists. The nature of the relationship with the provider; the degree to which the patient feels "safe" in confiding difficulties or concerns; the skill of the provider in eliciting patient perceptions; the extent to which a sense of partnership has been established regarding treatment decisions—all influence the patient's decision to re-contact providers and the degree to which medication-taking practices are reported and perceptions shared. Regardless of how completely patients report their experience with therapy (Box 1.2) when they re-contact providers, the provider will make a professional assessment of patient response to treatment based on what the patient does report and on lab values and other physiological measures. This assessment will lead to recommendations to continue drug treatment as previously recommended, to alter drug treatment (i.e., to change dose, change drug, add drug), or to discontinue drug treatment.

Analysis of the medication use process highlights several things. First, the decision by providers to advise or prescribe drug treatment is a small part of the process. Second, patients and professionals may be

---

Box 1.2 ENCOURAGE PATIENTS TO SHARE THEIR EXPERIENCE
WITH THERAPY

- They have unanswered questions.
- They have misunderstandings.
- They experience problems related to therapy.
- They "monitor" their own response to treatment.
- They make their own decisions regarding therapy.

AND

- They may not reveal this information to you unless **you** initiate a dialogue.

carrying out parallel decision-making with only sporadic communication about these processes. Furthermore, the communication that does occur may be incomplete and ineffective. Yet both patient and provider continue to make decisions and to evaluate outcomes, regardless of the quality of their understanding of each other's goals, actions, and decisions. One of the aims of the communication process should be to make the understanding of the patient and provider regarding the disease, illness experience, and treatment goals as congruent as possible.

It is obvious that there are numerous points in the process at which the quality of the patient–professional relationship and the thoroughness of the information exchange affect the decisions of both patients and health professionals. It is at these points that the communication skills of the professional are critical and can have the most effect on the outcomes of treatment.

SUMMARY

In establishing effective relationships with patients, the pharmacist must keep in mind his or her responsibility to help patients achieve desired health outcomes. The patient is the focus of the medication use process. The communication skills of pharmacists can facilitate formation of trusting relationships with patients. Pharmacists can establish an open exchange of information and foster a sense of partnership between patients and providers. An effective communication process can optimize the chance that patients will make informed decisions, use medications appropriately, and ultimately meet therapeutic goals.

REVIEW QUESTIONS

1. What is patient-centered care?
2. What does OBRA say about pharmacists' obligations?
3. What are the two primary functions that the communication process serves between health professionals and patients?
4. What is the benefit of analyzing the medication use process by patients?

References

Agency for Healthcare Research and Quality. 20 tips to help prevent medical errors. Patient Fact Sheet. AHRQ Publication No. 00-PO38 ed. Rockville, MD, 2000.

Beyth RJ, Quinn L, Landefeld CS. A multicomponent intervention to prevent major bleeding complications in older patients receiving warfarin: a randomized, controlled trial. *Annals of Internal Medicine* 133: 687–695, 2000.

Committee on Quality of Health Care in America, Institute of Medicine. *To err is human—building a safer health system.* Washington, DC, National Academy Press, 1999.

Conrad P. The meaning of medications: another look at compliance. *Social Science and Medicine* 20: 29–37, 1985.

Cox DJ, Gonder-Frederick L, Julian DM, Clarke W. Long-term follow-up evaluation of blood glucose awareness training. *Diabetes Care* 17: 1–5, 1994.

Cox DJ, Gonder-Frederick L, Polonsky W, et al. Blood glucose awareness training (BGAT-2): long-term benefits. *Diabetes Care* 24: 637–642, 2001.

Donovan JL, Blake DR. Patient non-compliance: deviance or reasoned decision-making? *Social Science and Medicine* 34: 507–513, 1992.

Ernst FR, Grizzle AJ. Drug-related morbidity and mortality: Updating the cost-of-illness model. *Journal of the American Pharmaceutical Association* 41: 192–199, 2001.

Greenfield S, Kaplan SH, Ware FE, Jr. Expanding patient involvement in care: effects on patient outcomes. *Annals of Internal Medicine* 102: 520–528, 1985.

Greenfield S, Kaplan SH, Ware JE, Jr. Patient participation in medical care: effects on blood sugar and quality of life in diabetes. *Journal of General Internal Medicine* 3: 448–457, 1988.

Hepler CD. Regulating for outcomes as a systems response to the problem of drug-related morbidity. *Journal of the American Pharmaceutical Association* 41: 108–115, 2001.

Hepler CD, Strand LM. Opportunities and responsibilities in pharmaceutical care. *American Journal of Hospital Pharmacy* 47: 533–543, 1990.

Hickson GB, Clayton EW, Githens PB, Sloan FA. Factors that prompted families to file medical malpractice claims following perinatal injuries. *JAMA* 267: 1359–1363, 1992.

Johnson JA , Bootman JL. Drug-related morbidity and mortality: a cost-of-illness model. *Archives of Internal Medicine* 155: 1949–1956, 1995.

Joint Commission on Accreditation of Healthcare Organizations (2002). Five steps to safer healthcare.

Kaplan SH, Greenfield S, Ware JE. Assessing the effects of physician-patient interactions on the outcomes of chronic disease. *Medical Care* 27: S110–S127, 1989.

Kimberlin C, Assa M, Rubin D, Zaenger P. Questions elderly patients have about on-going therapy: a pilot study to assist in communication with physicians. *Pharmacy World and Science* 23: 237–241, 2001.

Leape LL, Cullen DJ, Clapp MD, et al. Pharmacist participation on physician rounds and adverse drug events in the intensive care unit. *JAMA* 282: 267–270, 1999.

Manasse HR. Medication use in an imperfect world: drug misadventuring as an issue of public policy, part 1. *American Journal of Hospital Pharmacy* 46: 929–944, 1989.

Mead N, Bower P. Patient-centredness: a conceptual framework and review of the empirical literature. *Social Science and Medicine* 51: 1087–1110, 2000.

Roter DL. Patient question asking in physician-patient interaction. *Health Psychology* 3: 395–409, 1984.

Trostle JA. Medical compliance as an ideology. *Social Science and Medicine* 27: 1299–1308, 1988.

Part I
What Is
Communication?

Textbooks are written to answer three main questions: what, why, and how? This textbook is no different. It starts by answering the what- and why-type of questions: What is communication? Why is it important? It eventually addresses the how: How do I use these skills? How can I apply this to my own practice? Part I describes *what* is involved within communication: What are the key elements? What elements exist in pharmacist interactions with others? It serves as an introductory text for pharmacists and pharmacy students in the area of **interpersonal communication**, which can be described as one-to-one interaction between two individuals. Part I also addresses the important *why* questions: Why do I need to know this? Why is it important to pharmacy? Many of these elements may be obvious to the reader. However, as with any basic skill, the essential elements must first be examined before advancing to the application in practice settings. In addition, effective communication skills are necessary to build strong therapeutic relationships with patients.

The basic elements within interpersonal communication, including basic principles, the importance of perception, nonverbal aspects, and barriers to communication in pharmacy practice, are explored in Part I. The purpose is to encourage readers to examine their own communication skills and to pursue ways of improving their interpersonal skills with patients and their families, health care providers, and other pharmacy personnel. Examples and cases are provided to address the *how*-type of questions and to place these elements in the context of pharmacy practice. Although the book focuses on one-to-one interaction, many of these skills can be applied to group communication and to public speaking. The authors refer readers to comprehensive textbooks that deal with these other important areas of communication.

Chapter 2

Principles and Elements of Interpersonal Communication

■ OVERVIEW

Interpersonal communication is a common but complex practice that is essential in dealing with patients and other health care providers. This chapter describes the process of interpersonal communication as it relates to pharmacy practice and helps the reader determine what happens when one person tries to express an idea or exchange information with another individual. The information given here is the foundation for subsequent chapters that more fully describe ways of improving interpersonal relations and communication.

Setting the Stage

In our personal and professional lives, we all have to interact with other people. Some of these situations are successful; others are not. Consider the following situation:

> You are a pharmacist working alone in a community pharmacy. George Raymond, a 59-year-old man with moderate hypertension, enters the

pharmacy smoking a cigar. You know George because you attend the same church. He is a high school principal, has a wife who works, and has four children. He has been told to quit smoking and go on a diet. He also has a long history of not taking his medications correctly. He comes to pick up a new prescription—an antibiotic for a urinary tract infection. Although he knows you personally, he is somewhat hesitant as he approaches the prescription area. He looks down at the ground and mumbles, "The doctor called in a new prescription for me, and can I also have a refill of my heart medication?"

In most communication encounters, we typically do not have the opportunity to stop and analyze the situation. However, to improve our communication skills we need some ability to assess a particular situation quickly. Thus, for the situation just presented, take a moment now and on a sheet of paper briefly describe what Mr. Raymond might be thinking or feeling. What clues do you have? Write down what you might say to him. Set the paper aside and read on. Once you have finished the chapter, come back to your notes and rewrite your response based on any insights that resulted from your reading.

Components of the Interpersonal Communication Model

Communication encompasses a broad spectrum of media, for example, mass communication (TV, radio), small-group communication (committee meetings, discussion group), and large-group communication (lectures, speeches). This book focuses on one-to-one interpersonal communication that occurs in pharmacy practice, such as that observed in the situation with George Raymond. In this section, the interpersonal communication process, or the interaction between two individuals, will be described in detail. This specific form of communication (interpersonal communication) is best described as a process in which messages are generated and transmitted by one person and subsequently received and translated by another. A practical model of this process, as shown in Figure 2.1 combines five important elements: sender, message, receiver, feedback, and barriers.

The Sender

In the interpersonal communication process, the sender transmits a message to another person. In the example given, the initial sender of a message was Mr. Raymond.

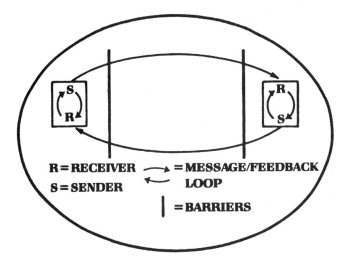

Figure 2.1   The interpersonal communication model.

The Message

In interpersonal communication, the message is the element that is transmitted from one person to another. Messages can be thoughts, ideas, emotions, information, or other factors and can be transmitted both verbally (by talking) and nonverbally (by using facial expressions, hand gestures, and so on). For example, Mr. Raymond's verbal message was that he wanted his new prescription and that he would like to have his prescription for heart medication refilled. At the same time, he also communicated nonverbal messages. Did you recognize any of these nonverbal messages? By looking down at the ground and mumbling rather than speaking clearly, he might have been expressing embarrassment, shyness, or hesitancy to talk with you. He might have felt embarrassed, perhaps because he had not been taking his heart pills regularly. As discussed in greater detail in Chapter 4, the nonverbal component of communication is important. Research has found that in some situations 55% or more of a message is transmitted through its nonverbal component.

In most situations, senders formulate or encode messages *before* transmitting them. However, in some cases, messages are transmitted spontaneously without the sender thinking about them, such as a glaring stare or a burst of laughter. In the earlier situation, Mr. Raymond may not have been aware that he was transmitting nonverbal messages to you.

The Receiver

The receiver (you, the pharmacist in the above example) receives the message from the sender (Mr. Raymond). As the receiver, you "decode" the message and assign a particular meaning to it, which may or may not be Mr. Raymond's intended meaning. In translating the message, you probably considered both the verbal and nonverbal components of the message.

Feedback

Feedback is the process whereby receivers communicate back to senders their understanding of the sender's message. In most situations, receivers do not passively absorb messages; they respond to them with their own verbal and nonverbal messages. By using verbal and nonverbal communication, the receiver feeds back information to the sender about how the message was translated. In the feedback loop, the initial receiver becomes the sender of feedback, and the initial sender becomes the receiver of feedback, as noted in the model. In the interpersonal communication process, individuals are thus constantly moving back and forth between the roles of sender and receiver. In the example, you were first a receiver of information; when you returned feedback to Mr. Raymond, you became a sender of information.

Feedback can be simple, such as merely nodding your head, or more complex, such as repeating a set of complicated instructions given to you to make sure that they were interpreted correctly. In the previous example, feedback would be your response to Mr. Raymond. On your paper, what did you indicate would be your response to Mr. Raymond? You could have said, "I'm sorry, George, I'm not sure what you are asking. Which medication do you need?" or "How are you feeling, George? You seem a bit down." Feedback allows communication to be a two-way process rather than a one-way monologue.

During the communication process, most of us tend to focus on the message and frequently miss the opportunity for feedback. As a receiver of a message, you may fail to provide appropriate feedback to the sender. As a sender of a message, you may fail to recognize feedback or to ask for feedback from the receiver. Consequently, you may be led to think that a communication interaction was more effective than it really was. As discussed in Chapter 6, being sensitive to others can strengthen our ability to receive and provide useful feedback.

Barriers

Interpersonal communication is usually affected by a number of interferences or barriers. These barriers affect the accuracy of the communication exchange. For example, if a loud vacuum cleaner was running in your pharmacy while you were talking to Mr. Raymond, it would have been even more difficult to understand what he was trying to communicate. Other physical barriers to your interaction with Mr. Raymond might include a safety glass partition between you and Mr. Raymond, telephones ringing in the background, or Mr. Raymond's defective hearing aid. Additional factors serving as barriers to communication are discussed in Chapter 5.

Responsibility of Pharmacists in the Communication Model

As a sender, you are responsible for ensuring that the message is transmitted in the clearest form, in terminology understood by the other person, and in an environment conducive to clear transmission. To check whether the message was received as intended, ask for feedback from the receiver and clarify any misunderstandings. Thus, your obligation as the sender of a message is not complete until you have determined that the other person has understood it correctly.

As a receiver, you have the responsibility of listening to what is transmitted by the sender. To ensure accurate communication, you should provide feedback to the sender by describing what you understood the message to be. Many times, we rely on our assumptions that we understand each other and thus feel that feedback is not necessary. However, research has found that without appropriate feedback, misunderstandings occur. Of concern is that, as pharmacists dealing with patients, physicians, and other health care providers, we cannot afford these misunderstandings. These misunderstandings might result in harm to the patient. To become more effective, efficient, and accurate in our communication, we must strive to include explicit feedback in our interactions with others.

In the roles of both receiver and sender, also be aware of the sources of interference or barriers to effective communication that exist and attempt to minimize them. Subsequent chapters illustrate ways to improve your skills as a receiver and a sender of messages. Ways to minimize communication barriers are also described.

In Search of the Meaning of the Message

The interpersonal communication model shows how messages originate from a sender and are received by a receiver. The sender delivers the message, and the receiver assigns a meaning to that message. The critical component in this process is that the receiver assigns the same meaning to the verbal or nonverbal message as intended by the sender. In other words, you may or may not interpret the message's meaning in the same way as the sender intended. In the encounter with Mr. Raymond, he may not have been embarrassed or hesitant to talk with you at all. He may have been looking down with dismay at a coffee stain on his new tie. He may have been upset at himself and was concentrating on his predicament rather than focusing on communicating clearly with you. Thus, the message that you received was not the one Mr. Raymond intended to send.

Words and Their Context

In general, individuals assign meaning to verbal and nonverbal messages based on their past experiences and previous definitions of these verbal and nonverbal elements. If two persons do not share the same definitions or past experiences, misunderstanding may occur. The most common example of this is evident in different languages and dialects of the world. Different words mean different things to different people based on the definitions learned. For example, "football" to an American means a sport using an oval ball, but "football" to a European means a sport using a round ball (soccer). An example of this misunderstanding occurs in health care when we speak in medical terminology that may have different (or possibly no) meaning to our patients. The following example illustrates this potential misunderstanding.

In the beginning exercise, let us assume that you wish to inform Mr. Raymond that his urinary tract antibiotic will be more effective if taken with sufficient fluid to guarantee adequate urinary output. You relate that intent in the following manner, "This medication should be taken with plenty of fluids." The message is received and decoded into words and symbols in the mind of Mr. Raymond. These words or symbols may or may not have any particular meaning to him. Perhaps he does not even know what "fluids" refers to; perhaps he is uncertain whether you consider milk to be a fluid; or perhaps he associates the word "plenty" with a small glass of orange juice at breakfast rather than the 8-ounce glass of water you had in mind. Thus, the meaning of your important message may or may not have been received accurately by Mr. Raymond. It is the assignment of meaning to those words by Mr. Raymond that is important.

Another important factor is that people assign meanings based on the context that they perceive the sender is using. Often patients understand the words that we are using but place them in a different context. Thus, they assign a meaning to our message that is different from the one intended. The following actual situation illustrates this point:

> A 9-month-old baby had to be admitted to the hospital with a severe infection due to the fact that his mother misunderstood the labeled instructions for an antibiotic: "Take one-half teaspoonful three times a

day for infection until all gone." The mother continued the drug for about three days until the baby appeared to be getting better. The mother then stopped giving the antibiotic; a superinfection developed; and the baby was hospitalized.

In this example, the mother interpreted the directions to mean "give the medication until the infection is all gone." The pharmacist intended to communicate that the medication (10 days' supply) should be continued until all the medication was gone. She understood the words used by the pharmacist, but she put them into a different context and thus derived a different meaning from the one intended by the pharmacist.

The social context also influences how messages are received and interpreted. The type of relationship that patients have with their pharmacists determines the level of acceptance that patients have regarding the information provided. Research has shown that if patients perceive pharmacists to be credible, unbiased providers of useful information, they will listen and retain more information about their medications. If they perceive pharmacists to be trustworthy and honest, they will be more willing to approach pharmacists for assistance.

Congruence Between Verbal and Nonverbal Messages

The meaning of the message may be somewhat unclear if the receiver senses incongruence between the verbal and nonverbal messages. That is, the meaning of a verbal message is not consistent with the meaning of a nonverbal message. The situations depicted in Box 2.1 reveal potentially incongruent messages.

In each of the previous examples, the verbal message obviously did

---

Box 2.1 EXAMPLES OF INCONGRUENT MESSAGES

- A beet-red-faced patron comes into the pharmacy, raises a fist, and loudly proclaims, "I'm not angry, I'm just here to ask about a prescription error."
- A disappointed pharmacist has tried for hours to convince a physician to change an obvious error in a patient's medication. When asked how he is feeling, he meekly replies, "Oh, I'm just fine."
- A patient hands a pharmacist a prescription for a tranquilizer, then bursts into tears. The pharmacist asks if anything is the matter, and the patient responds, "No, I'm okay, it's nothing at all."

not match the nonverbal message, and the receiver may be confused about the true message intended by the sender. To avoid this incongruence, as a sender you must be aware of the nonverbal messages as well as the verbal messages; as a receiver, you must point out to the sender that you are receiving two different messages.

In summary, people base their interpretation of verbal and nonverbal messages on a variety of factors. These factors include their definitions and perceptions of the words, symbols, and nonverbal elements used by the sender. The final message is not what is said, but what the receiver perceives was said. The following section discusses how to prevent potential misunderstandings.

Preventing Misunderstanding

In the previous situation involving the baby's antibiotic prescription, the label read, "Take one-half teaspoonful three times a day for infection until all gone." Unfortunately, the mother interpreted the message incorrectly. In this situation, the meaning could be clarified relatively easily by rearranging the position of the last two prepositional phrases (...three times a day until all gone for infection).

However, minimizing misunderstandings is many times more difficult in other situations. We often assume that the receiver will interpret our message accurately. We fail to realize that different people may assign different meanings to words or phrases that we use. We are generally unaware of this fact. To improve the communication process, we must remember that people assign meanings to messages based on their background, values, and experiences. If other persons have different backgrounds, values, and experiences, they may assign a different meaning to our intended message. Many of our problems in communication occur because we forget that individual experiences are never identical. In actual practice, we have enough common experiences with people we deal with on a daily basis that we can understand each other fairly well.

Typically, we can anticipate patients' feelings and their understanding about the use of drugs. Communication breaks down when we have limited common experiences or do not share the same meaning of certain words and symbols. Thus, a person placed on a medication for the first time has a different perception than a person who has taken the medication for several years; or a person of a different gender, age, or race may have experiences different from ours.

A key to preventing misunderstanding is anticipating how other people may translate your message. It may be helpful to determine their experience with drugs in general and with a particular drug specifically. If they have had positive experiences previously, their perception of drugs may be different than if they have had negative experiences. If they have negative feelings about drugs, then they may be reluctant to discuss the medication or even to take it. We need to ask certain questions to determine these perceptions. Have you been on this medication before? What have you heard about this medication? How do you feel about taking this medication? Some of the skills discussed in Chapter 6 on empathic listening may be helpful in anticipating how others may assign meaning to your message. In many communication interactions, the more you know about other people and the more you are able to understand them, the easier it will be to anticipate how they may interpret the meaning of the message.

Using Feedback to Check the Meaning of the Message

Predicting how a person will translate a particular message is difficult. Using a technique described earlier (providing feedback to check the meaning of the message) may alleviate some communication misunderstandings. As senders of messages, we should ask others to share their interpretation of the message. In the example of the antibiotic, the pharmacist should have asked the mother in a nonthreatening manner, "When you get home, how long are you going to give the medication?" We typically do not ask for feedback from patrons to check their perceptions of the meaning of our messages. Verifying the fact that the receiver interpreted the intended meaning of our verbal and nonverbal messages accurately takes additional time and is sometimes awkward. Most people rely on their own intuition as to whether their intended message was received correctly. Unfortunately, relying on our intuition is not as effective as obtaining explicit feedback to measure understanding.

In the antibiotic example, the pharmacist who dispensed the original medication should have asked the mother how she intended to give the medication to her baby and how long she would continue to give the baby the medicine. Thus, her initial perception could have been corrected, and the problem could have been avoided. Examples of how to ask for feedback are shown in Box 2.2.

The preceding paragraphs describe ways to minimize misunderstanding from the sender's perspective. However, the receiver can also alleviate some misunderstanding by offering feedback to the sender. After receiving the message, the receiver should indicate in some way what she understands the message to be. In later chapters, specific skills are offered as means of improving your ability to give feedback and receive feedback from others.

Box 2.2 STATEMENTS OR QUESTIONS THAT ELICIT FEEDBACK

- "I want to be sure I have explained things clearly. Please summarize the most important things to remember about this medicine."
- "How do you intend to take the medication?"
- "Please show me how you are going to use this nasal inhaler."
- "It is important that I understand that you know how to take this medication. Now when you get home, how are you going to take this medication?"
- "Describe in your own words how you are going to take this medication."

Improving Communication Behaviors

This chapter has presented elements of interpersonal communication and outlined strategies to improve communication skills. The discussion of improvement implies that behaviors that inhibit communication must be altered. When attempting to change communication behaviors, it is important to place these potential behavioral changes in relation to two other concepts: awareness and attitude. As illustrated by Figure 2.2, a change in behavior is frequently built on appropriate awareness and attitudes that are conducive to potential behavior change.

If you hope to develop new behavior, you must increase awareness of your present behavior and also change your attitude toward interacting with others. Awareness of the communication process centers on two important concepts: self awareness and process awareness.

Self-awareness is the process of recognizing how you actually communicate with others using both verbal and nonverbal messages. It is the process of analyzing how you are communicating at the actual time

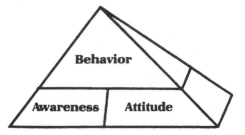

Figure 2.2 A model for improving communication.

of the interaction. Part of this process is asking questions such as "What type of nonverbal messages am I sending?" and "Am I using the correct terminology for this patient?"

To enhance their own self-awareness, many pharmacists videotape themselves in simulated or actual practice settings. Some pharmacists have colleagues, administrators, or faculty critique their performance. This process makes them aware of their strengths and weaknesses in this important area.

Process awareness involves analyzing the communication process itself while it is occurring. You have to ask yourself, "Is the conversation going in the direction it should go?" "Am I talking too much?" "Are we getting sidetracked?" If the interaction is not proceeding in the desired direction, then you must tactfully move the interaction toward that direction by using some of the communication skills discussed in this book.

Changing behavior is very difficult in most situations. People have difficulty in changing how they take medications or how they communicate with others. However, as revealed in Chapter 9, strategies exist that help people plan for and implement change. As pharmacists, we must review our present communication behavior and at the same time develop an attitude that improved communication is important. Effective communication techniques yield better patient rapport, more accurate information, optimal patient therapies, greater job satisfaction, and efficiencies arising from better understanding.

SUMMARY

The interpersonal communication model reveals that, as a pharmacist, you must recognize that interpersonal communication is more than merely speaking to others, typing a prescription label, or affixing an auxiliary label to a prescription. You must make sure that the messages you transmit to others are received accurately. There is no guarantee that the meaning of your message will be translated as intended. You need to make sure that you enhance your listening skills so that you can become a better receiver of messages as well.

In the remaining chapters, we provide practical skills necessary for improving your communication. Each chapter builds on the preceding one. Communication is a complex process that may be difficult for some. However, it is a process that can be easily managed and controlled like any other learned skill. By emphasizing practical applications, we hope to lower any barriers that you may have to improvement of the valuable skills involved in communicating effectively. Before going further, go back and reread your comments about Mr. Raymond's situation and change anything that you would do differently.

REVIEW QUESTIONS

1. Describe the five components in the communications model.
2. Where do the meanings of messages come from?
3. What happens when verbal and nonverbal messages are not congruent?
4. How can misperceptions be minimized?

SUGGESTED READINGS

Adler AR. *Communicating at Work*. New York: Random House, 1986.

Beebe SA, Beebe SJ, Redmond MV. *Interpersonal Communication: Relating to Others*. 2nd ed. Boston: Allyn & Bacon, 1999.

Berko RM, Wolvin AD, Wolvin DR. *Communicating: A Social and Career Focus*. Boston: Houghton Mifflin, 1989.

Borman EG, Borman NC. *Effective Small Group Communication*. Minneapolis: Gordon Press, 1986.

Burnard P. *Communicate!: A Communication Skills Guide for Health Care Workers*. London: E. Arnold, 1992.

Casswell HD. The structure and function of communication in society. In L. Bryson, ed. *The Communication of Ideas*. New York: Institute for Religion and Social Studies, 1948.

Eriksen K. *Communication Skills for the Human Services*. Reston, VA: Reston Publishing Company, 1979.

Hargie OD, Morrow NC, Woodman C. Pharmacists' evaluation of key communication skills in practice. *Patient Education and Counseling* 39: 61-70, 2000.

Taylor A, Rose Grant T, Mayer A, Samples BT. *Communications,* 4th ed. Englewood Cliffs, NJ: Prentice-Hall, 1986.

Ver Derber RS, Ver Derber KS. *Interact: Using Interpersonal Communication Skills*. Belmont, CA: Wadsworth, 1989.

Wood JT. *Interpersonal Communication-Everyday Encounters,* 2nd ed. New York: Wadsworth, 1999.

Chapter 3

Perception in Professional Communication

Perception of Meanings in a Message

Perceptions of Individuals

Sharing the Same Perceptions

Using Feedback to Verify Perceptions

Perception, Credibility, and Persuasion

▨ OVERVIEW

Perception is important in the process of interpersonal communication because people interpret messages based on their perception of (a) what they believe the message says and (b) the individual sending the message. Thus, perceptual barriers exist in all of us and need to be minimized or we will misunderstand what we hear. Two skills for pharmacists that help reduce misperceptions are to always recognize how fragile the communication process is during professional communication and to use feedback to enhance our ability to verify the true meaning of messages.

Perception of Meanings in a Message

People assign meaning to verbal and nonverbal messages based on their perception of the intended meaning (Fabun, 1986). In other words, the receiver's perception of the words, symbols, and nonverbal elements used by the sender influences how the receiver interprets the meaning. It is not what is said, but what the receiver perceives to have been said. The following actual situation illustrates this point.

A patient returned to the pharmacy complaining of side effects apparently caused by his medication. The patient's records indicated he was given 30 nitroglycerin patches. Both the pharmacist and the physician told him to "apply one daily." The patient opened his shirt to reveal that 27 nitroglycerin patches were firmly adhered to his chest. He perceived that the phrase "apply one daily" was an absolute, and because no one asked him for feedback on the directions, he applied them, (but did not remove them) as he perceived the instructions to be. A little time spent with him verifying his understanding would have saved him embarrassment and distressing side effects.

Misperceptions like the latter occur frequently in pharmacy practice, and every pharmacist has a story to tell. The outcome of such misperception may be relatively harmless, but some can be serious. For example:

A young woman suffering vaginal candidiasis was given the usual 15 nystatin vaginal tablets and was told by the pharmacist to "use one daily for two weeks." She returned to her physician after two weeks in severe discomfort with a complaint that "those tablets taste terrible!" In this example, the patient perceived the tablets as being nothing more than regular oral antibiotics and assigned a wrong meaning to the word "use."

Preventing incorrect perceptions is often difficult because people with whom you interact may have different perceptions about the messages you transmit. Unfortunately, these differences may influence how they interpret messages. In general, people develop their perceptions based on their background, values, and experiences. People of different backgrounds, values, and experiences may assign meanings to messages that are different from the meanings intended by the sender. We are generally unaware of this process, and it takes skill to realize when we have different perceptions from those with whom we are trying to communicate.

It is a very easy matter to have patients misunderstand what a pharmacist has instructed them to do, especially when the pharmacist uses language that is overly abstract. Instructions that are abstract but in common use include: "Drink a lot of fluid" or "Take this as your doctor instructed." Such broad, nonspecific directions raise more questions than they provide answers. To prevent misperceptions and misunderstandings, pharmacists can keep the following in mind:

1. Avoid the use of equivocal terms, that is, words with more than one meaning.
2. Avoid use of professional jargon. This advice is especially true when professionals deal with culturally diverse populations for whom "plain talk" always works best. For example, most people are not impressed by the fact that a pharmacist knows they have intermittent claudication, when what they want is help with their inability to walk any distance without experiencing leg pain.

3. Use low-level abstractions to build clarity. Any idea can be expressed using various levels of abstractions. But when it comes to illness and medicines, simple ideas and words are the most helpful. For example, ask someone to "describe your pain on a scale of 0 to 10 with '0' being no pain and '10' being the worst pain imaginable." This will be more helpful than asking someone, "does it hurt a lot?"

4. Recognize the differences in cross-cultural styles of speaking. Much research has been done in the past decade on this and on the differences in the ways that men and women converse. Although the popular press makes great note of such work, these differences are not absolutes, especially in professions in which the roles of men and women have become less distinct. For more on this read the work of Deborah Tannen (1994) who says that women talk more to (a) establish connections, (b) establish good will, (c) show support, and (d) establish community, whereas men tend to talk in a style that (a) focuses on the task at hand, (b) focuses on reporting, and (c) focuses on asserting control over the situation.

Perceptions of Individuals

Our perception of the message is also influenced by our perception of the individual sending the message (Keltner, 1970). How we perceive the sender affects the interpretation of the message. We respond using our perception of that individual as our reference point because we tend to be influenced by a person's cultural background, socioeconomic status, gender, or age. These perceptions are further influenced by any bias we have or stereotypes we hold of certain groups of individuals. The following statements illustrate this point.

"People who are mentally ill do not comply with their medication regimens."
"Nurses always complain about pharmacists."
"Elderly people can't hear well and always talk too much."
"People who talk slow are lazy."
"Women with red hair have a temper."
"People who are overweight are jolly."

We do not see the person as a unique individual but as a representative of a particular group (e.g., elderly, overweight, or mentally ill). We erect "perceptual barriers" to the communication process not based on fact but on our inferences based on stereotypes. These barriers inhibit true communication between individuals.

It is important to realize that in our normal interactions with others we create perceptions of individuals and make various assumptions. For example, we tend to believe that our patients can speak and understand English well enough to understand us unless they tell us otherwise. Unfortunately, this is not always the case because many patients, in an effort to avoid embarrassment, do not indicate that they do not understand our instructions. We need to evaluate when our perception of the sender is incorrect or when our assumptions might be interfering with our ability to communicate with others. We may need to "check" our assumption before proceeding. Does the elderly person really have a hearing deficiency? Does the person who talks slowly have a learning disability? Increased awareness of stereotyping and additional effort in checking our assumptions can enhance our interpersonal communication.

Unfortunately, people we deal with on a daily basis may have perceptions of pharmacists that interfere with our ability to communicate with them. Their perceptions may not be based on reality but on their stereotypes of pharmacists. Patient perceptions are influenced by their past experiences with pharmacists, by what others have said about pharmacists, or by what they read in magazines and newspapers. For example, patients may perceive us as uncaring, busy people who are concerned only with filling prescriptions and taking their money. These stereotypes influence what they say to us and how they listen to us. If they perceive us as professionals, they will listen to what we tell them about their medications. By the same token, if nurses, physicians, and other health care providers do not perceive us as professionals, they will not value the information we provide. Part of improving communication with others is to determine what their perceptions of pharmacists are and then try to alter those perceptions if they are unfounded.

Sharing the Same Perceptions

One key to preventing misunderstanding is to try to understand and share the perceptions of other individuals (Applebaum et al, 1985). Many times, using "lay language," which is familiar to patients, rather than medical terminology, which is familiar only to health care professionals, can enhance understanding. Determining the patient's past experience with medications or with the particular drugs prescribed may also be helpful. Patients who have had positive experiences previously may be more willing to take the medication. However, if their past experiences have been bad, they may be reluctant to even begin taking the medication.

Frequently, it is difficult to understand patient backgrounds and to predict perceptions of the messages we provide (Box 3.1). Some of the skills discussed in Chapter 6 on empathic listening may be helpful. In many communication interactions, the more we can know about the other person and the more they can know about us, the easier it is to

Box 3.1 ADVICE PHARMACISTS SHOULD FOLLOW WHEN
COMMUNICATING WITH PEOPLE OF DIFFERENT
BACKGROUNDS

- Learn as much as you can about other cultures. Most communication problems arise when there is a lack of knowledge about
  the other person's reasons for a particular communication style.
- View diversity as an opportunity. With a little patience and the
  right attitude, you will be amazed at the opportunities that crop
  up to help one another.
- Do not condescend. Patronizing behavior is not appreciated and
  is recognized as such in any culture.
- Talk about your differences. Misunderstandings will often take
  root when people from differing backgrounds do not talk to one
  another. Be willing to talk openly and with a constructive attitude

share the same perception. In past generations, most pharmacists could
spend their entire lives in a career that rarely caused them to encounter
people from different backgrounds. Today, cultural diversity is a fact of
life throughout America. In fact, a culturally diverse workplace has
become the norm. It shapes the way people communicate because communication is something learned rather than something innate.
Pharmacists, as members of the helping professions, know that when
they stop to talk and genuinely listen, sometimes even the smallest of
efforts can make a miracle happen.

Using Feedback to Verify Perceptions

The best technique to alleviate communication misunderstandings is
through feedback, because this will help to verify the perceived meaning of a message. As senders of messages, we should ask others to share
their interpretations of the message. In the nitroglycerin example, the
pharmacist should have asked the patient in a nonthreatening manner
how he was going to use the patches. We typically do not ask for feedback from patients to check their perceptions of the words used when
we give directions. We simply assume that patients understand us. Just
think how many medication misadventures could be prevented if pharmacists would ask patients to give them feedback using this phrase,
"Before you leave could you please tell me how you are going to use
this medicine?"

The receiver can also alleviate some misunderstanding by offering
feedback to the sender. After receiving the message, receivers should
summarize the key elements of the message. In later chapters, specific

A patient, Ms. Reynolds, enters a pharmacy having just come from her physician's office.

> *Ms. Reynolds: My doctor just gave me a prescription for Methotrexate and did not tell me anything about it!! What's it used for?*
> *Pharmacist: I am kind of busy right now to go into detail, but it is used to treat cancer.*
> *Ms. Reynolds: What?!! Oh my goodness!! I can't believe this. I'm not going to take this stuff—it will probably make me feel even worse.*

How could have the pharmacist handled this situation differently to check for misperceptions?

What would you have said to the patient?

Would you call anyone else about this? If so, who?

skills are offered to improve our ability to give feedback and receive feedback from others.

Perception, Credibility, and Persuasion

In many situations, pharmacists must try to influence the decisions of patients, physicians, and others. The pharmacist may need to convince a patient that he must take the full 10-day course of antibiotics. Or, the pharmacist may want to convince a Pharmacy & Therapeutics Committee in a hospital to delete a certain drug from the formulary. In the search to find the variable that makes one person more persuasive than another, research points to only one factor—perceived credibility. People are influenced by individuals they believe to be credible. Being perceived as credible will enhance the pharmacist's ability to be persuasive more effectively than spending hours polishing an impressive style.

What constitutes the perception of credibility? There is agreement that perceived credibility is the combination of three factors:

1. A safety or trustworthiness element
2. An expertness or qualifications element
3. A personal or dynamism element

The *trustworthiness* factor is a subjective response to the warmth, friendliness, ethics, sociability, fairness, and other things that enhance

REVIEW CASE 3.2

You are a pharmacist in a pharmacy located in a medical building. Cynthia Jackson, a 22-year-old college student, enters your pharmacy. Cynthia has no prescription insurance and is on a limited budget. She has been dealing with chronic sinusitis and finally realized that she needed to see an ear, nose, and throat specialist. Cynthia visited Dr. Sampson, who practices in your building. You know Dr. Sampson to be a good physician, but one who lacks interpersonal skills at times. He prescribed an expensive antibiotic that would cost Cynthia $75. After you tell her the price, Cynthia states:

> That darn Dr. Sampson didn't help me very much. He spends 5 minutes with me and then prescribes this expensive antibiotic and nothing else! And how do you get off charging me so much for that stupid antibiotic?

What feelings do you sense coming from Cynthia?

How does Cynthia's perception of Dr. Sampson influence her behavior?

How would you respond to Cynthia?

What kind of recommendations would you give her?

---

the perception of someone being "safe" to talk to. This element is important even when conversation requires little or no expertise. Thus, pharmacists who are trusted may find patients asking advice on non-health matters such as personal finance, relationships, buying a car, choosing a college, or any number of subjects.

The *expertness* factor involves a perception about the competence or education of a sender. It is a factor independent of the other two. One can be labeled trustworthy and highly personable, but sadly lacking in expertise. Naturally, we wish to be perceived as competent by all those who seek our advice. Since the public will subjectively evaluate any and all behavior that relates to competency, we should engage in activities that promote competence, such as displaying awards, certificates, diplomas, and licenses; giving public service talks when asked; seeking and holding office in professional societies; and taking every opportunity to explain what it is that makes a pharmacist a valued member of society.

The *personal dynamism* factor relates to overall personal characteristics of the sender as perceived by the receiver. For instance, if a pharmacist who counsels a patient for the first time happens to stumble over administration instructions, is slow to respond, and is quite shy, then that pharmacist's credibility may be ranked low despite his great credentials and extensive knowledge base. However, as subsequent interviews occur, initial judgments may fade if the pharmacist can demonstrate trustworthiness and expertness after the patient gets to know him or her. In reality, our interpersonal credibility results from the perception that our clientele has of our trustworthiness, competence, and personal dynamism combined. Before reading further, pause for a moment and ask yourself the following:

1. How do I believe my patients perceive my credibility?
2. What can I do if I believe my trustworthiness or competence is rated low?
3. Do I have any personal traits or habits that keep my patients from getting to perceive the "real" me?

SUMMARY

The meaning of the message is influenced by the receiver's perception of the intended message and of the individual sending the message. The following saying summarizes this dilemma: "I know that you believe you understand what you think I said, but I'm not sure you realize what you heard is not what I meant." Thus, it is important to remember the following points when communicating with others:

1. Anticipate different perceptions in the communication process.
2. Try to be aware of stereotypes you hold that may influence your perception of others and also be aware of stereotypes others may have of you.
3. Ask for feedback from the receiver about how well your intended message was received.
4. Provide feedback to the sender to check your perception of the message and to make sure you understood correctly.
5. Evaluate your level of trustworthiness, competence, and personal dynamism as perceived by others.

REVIEW QUESTIONS

1. How do perceptions interfere with communications?
2. What is meant by "Our perception of a message is affected by our perception of the individual?"
3. What are two ways you can prevent perceptual misunderstandings?
4. Why is it important to ask for feedback?

References

Applebaum RL, Jenson DO, Caroll R. *Speech Communication*. New York: Macmillan, 1985.

Fabun D. *Communications: The Transfer of Meaning*. Toronto: Glencoe Press, 1986.

Keltner SW. *Interpersonal Speech Communication: Elements and Structures*. Belmont, CA: Wadsworth, 1970.

Tannen D. *Talking from 9–5*. New York: Morrow, 1994.

Chapter 4

Nonverbal Communication in Pharmacy

Nonverbal versus Verbal Communication

Elements of Nonverbal Communication

Distracting Nonverbal Communication

Detecting Nonverbal Cues in Others

Overcoming Distracting Nonverbal Factors

■ OVERVIEW

Words are not the only way in which pharmacists communicate. Interpersonal communication involves both verbal and nonverbal expression. Words normally express ideas, whereas nonverbal expressions convey attitudes and emotions. Nonverbal expressions include kinesics, proxemics, and the physical environment in which communication takes place. A large measure of how you relate to others and how they relate to you is not based on what is said, but on what is not said. You may not speak or even have the desire to communicate and yet be engaged in a communication process. You are constantly providing "messages" to those around you by your dress, facial expression, body movements, and other aspects of your appearance and behavior. This chapter introduces nonverbal communication and discusses how it plays an important role in effective patient-centered communication.

Nonverbal versus Verbal Communication

Nonverbal communication involves a complete mix of behaviors, psychological responses, and environmental interactions through which a person consciously and unconsciously relates to another person. It differs from verbal communication in that the medium of exchange is neither vocalized language nor the written word. The importance of nonverbal communication is underlined by the findings of behavioral scientists, which have reported that approximately 55% to 95% of all communication can be attributed to nonverbal sources (Mehrabian, 1971; Poytos, 1983). Awareness and skilled use of your nonverbal abilities can make the difference between fulfilling, successful interpersonal relations and frustrated, nonproductive interactions.

Nonverbal communications are unique for two reasons. First, they mirror innermost thoughts and feelings. This mirror effect is constantly at work, whether or not you are conscious of it. Second, nonverbal communication is difficult, if not impossible, to "fake" during an interpersonal interaction. Lack of congruence between your verbal and nonverbal messages may result in less than successful interpersonal communication (Borman et al, 1969).

In nonverbal communication, each person perceives and interprets a given nonverbal message or "cue" in a personal manner. Various interpretations emerge from the different social, psychological, cultural, and other background variables of the senders and receivers of nonverbal messages. For example, a simple nod of the head may mean something to one person but something completely different to another. Therefore, nonverbal "cues" can and often do have multiple interpretations. However, within a given society, groups of nonverbal cues or "cue clusters" generally result in interpretations that are usually universally agreed upon.

Cue clusters are combinations of nonverbal acts that communicate certain global messages. For example, a patient who gives you a friendly handshake, a pleasant-sounding "thank you," and a warm smile at the end of your interaction is probably more pleased with the interaction than a patient who abruptly turns around and quickly walks away mumbling something under his breath. Without a doubt, cue clusters contribute significantly to what is being communicated nonverbally. On the other hand, the specific "reasons" behind a person's nonverbal behaviors, for example "why" a patient turned abruptly and walked away, usually cannot be determined from the nonverbal communication alone. You can know that the patient seems upset. However, you cannot know whether the cause is distress over something you said, discouragement at being ill, dismay over the cost of the medication, hurry to get back to work, or myriad other things that may be on the patient's mind and explain his or her behavior. When analyzing nonverbal communication, avoid focusing on just one cue, but look at all the nonverbal cues that you are receiving and use verbal communication to fully understand the meaning of the nonverbal behavior.

> **Box 4.1** ELEMENTS OF NONVERBAL COMMUNICATION
>
> - Kinesics
> - Proxemics
> - Environment
> - Distracting factors

Elements of Nonverbal Communication

Important nonverbal elements discussed here include kinesics, or body movement; proxemics, or the distance between persons when they communicate; the physical environment; and potential distracting nonverbal elements (Box 4.1).

Kinesics

The manner in which you use your arms, legs, hands, head, face, and torso may have a dramatic impact on the messages that you send. Societies have developed and use numerous body movements to communicate certain messages. In this country, for example, it is common for two men to shake hands when meeting each other. A handshake is a way by which we nonverbally indicate friendship or acceptance of another person. The handshake stems from much earlier times, when a man who extended his hand to another was communicating the fact that he held no weapon to do harm to the other. Many of our common nonverbal acts stem from earlier times. And so current meanings of many of these acts may bear little resemblance to their initial meanings.

As a health care professional, you need to generate a feeling of empathy and commitment to the helping of others. It is apparent, therefore, that your body movement or *kinesics* should complement this role. An open stance can nonverbally communicate sincerity, respect, and empathy for another person. The classic example of an open posture is standing (or sitting) with a full frontal appearance to the other person. As an open communicator, you should also have your legs comfortably apart (not crossed), arms uncrossed, and a facial expression that expresses interest and a desire to listen as well as speak.

A closed posture, one that would not lend itself to continued communication, occurs when you have your arms folded in front of your chest, legs crossed at the knees, head facing downward, and eyes looking at the floor. If you hold this posture during the interaction, the other person may either respond in a similar manner or break off the interaction. Communication from a closed posture may shorten or halt further productive interaction. Sometimes it is appropriate to use a closed posture. For example, when you want to limit the interaction with an

> **Box 4.2** KEY COMPONENTS OF KINESICS
>
> - Varied eye contact (consistent, but not a stare)
> - Relaxed posture
> - Appropriate comfortable gestures
> - Frontal appearance (shoulders square to other person)
> - Slight lean toward the other person
> - Erect body position (head up, shoulders back)

overly talkative salesperson, you may assume a closed posture to discourage continued conversation.

The key is to be aware of your tendency to close off communication through your nonverbal communication. For example, if during a consultation you suddenly have the impression that the patient is no longer interested in speaking with you, examine your nonverbal communication to see if it has caused ill feelings. To improve communication kinesics, consider the suggestions in Box 4.2.

Proxemics

The distance between two interacting persons plays an important role in the message that is communicated. *Proxemics*, the structure and use of space, is a powerful nonverbal communication tool. Behavioral scientists have found that at different distances between communicators different communications normally transpire (Keltner, 1970). The most protected space is that from full contact to approximately 18 inches from our bodies. We reserve this space for others with whom we have close, intimate relationships. When a stranger, or even a non-intimate associate, ventures into this space during a conversation, we experience anxiety and perhaps anger at the trespass of our intimate zone. A crowded elevator is the best illustration of our need to maintain our intimate space. People in a crowded elevator will do almost anything (to the point of standing like statues) to avoid touching one another. If by chance two people in this situation do have bodily contact, they usually make profuse apologies, even though neither person may have had an opportunity to avoid the trespass of space.

We are much more comfortable in our daily interactions when we maintain a distance of 18 inches to 48 inches between other individuals. At this distance, casual personal conversations normally take place. In pharmacy practice, most interactions occur when both parties are about 4 to 12 feet from each other. Interpersonal distances of more than

12 feet are generally reserved for occasions when one person is speaking to a group. This distance would not be appropriate for private conversations.

You may want to consider the factor of distance whenever you consult with patients. When counseling a patient, it is important to stand close enough to ensure privacy, yet at the same time to provide enough room for each person to feel comfortable. You do not want to invade a patient's intimate zone. Patients usually indicate nonverbally whether they feel comfortable with the speaking distance by stepping back or leaning forward.

You should also be aware of interacting at distances that are inappropriate for the nature of the conversation. If you attempt to explain the usage of a rectal or vaginal medication at a public distance you risk embarrassing the patient. Ideally, the pharmacy should provide appropriate levels of privacy so that both the sender and the receiver of messages feel comfortable.

Environmental Nonverbal Factors

A number of environmental factors play an important role in communicating nonverbal messages to patients. For example, a private consulting area could aid communication by providing the appropriate distance between you and your patients. The colors used in the pharmacy's decor, the lighting, and the uses of space in the pharmacy all have been documented as important nonverbal communication factors (Beardsley et al, 1977). How you use the prescription counter is an important environmental factor. The counter and related shelving serve to keep the prescription dispensing somewhat private from the public. However, it can certainly serve as a barrier to communication if it inhibits your ability to counsel patients effectively. Although the prescription counter serves a utilitarian purpose, it should not be seen as the Great Wall of China. When appropriate, step from behind the counter to communicate a genuine interest in talking with patients about their medications.

The general appearance of the pharmacy also plays an important role in conveying nonverbally that you are a professional and that you are sincerely interested in serving your patrons. Dirt, clutter, and general untidiness in any business carry a negative nonverbal message. In addition, physical characteristics of pharmacy employees also send nonverbal messages. Professional staff should dress appropriately. You want to convey a friendly appearance, but you also want to convey professional competence. Your appearance and the appearance of your fellow employees can complement or destroy other nonverbal efforts to communicate professionalism.

Distracting Nonverbal Communication

As discussed in Chapter 2, communication is the transmission of both nonverbal and verbal messages in an environment plagued with barriers. An initial step in improving the communication process is to become more aware of these barriers. Some of the more common nonverbal barriers are discussed in the following text.

One of the most obvious barriers in nonverbal communication is lack of eye contact with the patient. It is frustrating to talk to somebody who is not looking at you. Unfortunately, many pharmacists unconsciously do not look at patients when talking to them. Their tendency is to look at the prescription, the prescription container, or other objects while talking. This behavior could indicate to patients that you are not really confident about what you are saying or that you do not really care about the patient. Not looking at the patient also limits your ability to assess how the information you are providing is affecting that person. In other words, lack of eye contact limits your ability to receive feedback from the patient. For instance, does the patient have a questioning look, an expression of surprise, an expression of contentment? As discussed in Chapter 6, good eye contact is essential to effective listening. If you do not look patients in the eye, they may get the impression that you are not interested in what they are saying; thus, they might not feel comfortable communicating with you. Using good eye contact does not actually mean that you continually stare at patients, but that you spend most of the time looking at them.

Another potentially distracting nonverbal element is facial expression. You may be sending a message that you did not intend to transmit. For example, if your eyes continue to move around while talking or listening to another person, you may be communicating a feeling of lack of interest or concern. This is especially damaging when your facial expressions are not consistent with your verbal expressions. For example, if you say to someone, "Go ahead I am listening, tell me about it." Then you appear to be distracted by something else around you, the person may hear you say that you are interested, but may perceive that you are not by observing your nonverbal communication. People tend to believe your facial messages more than the verbal aspects of the communication.

In addition to facial expression, body position in relation to the patient can show a lack of concern or interest. That is, whether you are positioned in an open or closed stance communicates either concern or lack of interest. Your body position is also determined by whether you fold your arms, slouch forward, or tilt to one side. Patients read or sense your willingness to talk to them based on their perception of your body position, which can communicate whether you are really prepared to talk with them or you have more important things to do.

Another potential distraction to communication is your tone of voice. People interpret the message not only by the words you use, but also by the tone of voice you use. For example, a comment in a sarcastic or threatening tone of voice will produce a different effect than the same phrase spoken with an empathic tone. Conveying a message in a monotone voice may convey a lack of interest in the communication. An inappropriate tone of voice can upset people and may create an entirely different meaning from the one intended. To remove this potential barrier, many pharmacists have recorded their voices to monitor inflection and its effect on communication. And many have found that they sound far different from what they expected.

The manner in which you use time also conveys a number of silent messages (McGrath and Kelsey, 1989). If you keep physicians' offices waiting on the telephone, do not acknowledge customers waiting in a line, or cut a counseling session short to answer the phone, you are sending nonverbal messages that your time is more valuable than that of others.

Detecting Nonverbal Clues in Others

Up to this point, attention has been focused on assessing your own nonverbal communication. Understanding nonverbal communication also involves detecting the nonverbal cues provided by others. It would be impossible to list all the potential nonverbal cues that you could observe from the patients. Assessing the meaning behind the nonverbal communication of others is difficult, because we interpret nonverbal cues based on our personal backgrounds and experiences. The key is to be aware of these differences so as not to make false assumptions or jump to conclusions based on your interpretation of nonverbal cues.

Some elderly and physically ill persons may have limited or impaired sense capabilities that will influence how they communicate nonverbally. Thus, you need to adjust your communication in accordance with the messages these nonverbal cues are sending you. For example, elderly patients may move closer to you or may put a hand to their ears. This may indicate that they are having difficulty in hearing. You may also observe hearing aids, glasses, and other devices that may indicate possible communication barriers.

As part of the detection process, check your perception of nonverbal messages, since the messages that you receive may not be the messages intended by the sender. The following example illustrates this point.

During his first externship experience in a community pharmacy, a pharmacy student (John) was assigned the task of receiving new prescriptions from patients. John wanted to help the patients and was looking forward to the opportunity of talking with them about their problems. One day, Mr. Stevens approached the prescription counter to have his prescription for levodopa refilled. John, who did not realize that Mr. Stevens had Parkinson's disease, noticed that his hands were shaking and commented, "I see you are a bit nervous today, Mr. Stevens. What's the matter?" John observed a nonverbal message (rapid hand movement) from Mr. Stevens and assigned a wrong (and embarrassing) meaning to it. John should not have jumped to the conclusion based on one nonverbal cue but should have noticed that Mr. Stevens' head was also moving and that he walked with a shuffled gait characteristic of Parkinson's disease.

Dealing with Sensitive Issues

A Harris Survey (Harris, 1997) found that the most common reason consumers do not seek medical attention is embarrassment. From the patient's standpoint, embarrassing problems include a wide variety of conditions, such as incontinence, sexual dysfunction, depression, menopause, hemorrhoids, contraception, and breast or prostate cancer.

As a pharmacist, you should be prepared to recognize situations that may lead to possible patient embarrassment. You should be comfortable discussing such matters in a nonthreatening way and in a nonverbal environment that conveys confidentiality and privacy. Here are some tips and tactics to help with such situations.

1. Watch your patients. Before engaging in a conversation, watch their behavior to get a clue about their feelings. They may appear to be embarrassed before they reach the prescription counter.

2. Discuss sensitive issues with clarity and avoid potentially frightening scenarios. For example, you may bring up the subject of incontinence by saying, "Miss Smith, we have many women who get their prescriptions from us here for bladder control problems. While this problem is potentially embarrassing, there are several effective means to deal with it. Would you like to step away to a more quiet area and we can discuss it?"

3. Be cognizant of the potential for nonadherence. Many patients with embarrassing conditions do not follow their medical regimens as directed. Check medication refill rates and observe patients' behavior when they are describing how they take their medications. If you suspect nonadherence to medication regimens, ask open-ended questions to assess patient attitudes and feelings. For example, you could ask "How do you feel about taking this medication?" This gives you an opportunity to watch and listen to both verbal and nonverbal messages.

Overcoming Distracting Nonverbal Factors

As mentioned earlier, the first step in improving interpersonal communication is recognizing how you communicate with others. In the nonverbal area, this self-awareness involves being constantly aware of your nonverbal behavior. In this regard, videotaping yourself is particularly helpful, since it reveals the positive and negative aspects of your nonverbal communication.

Once you have discovered what aspects you need to change to become more effective, the next step is a difficult one: finding strategies to overcome these distracting elements. Several suggestions have been already made about how specific nonverbal elements can be improved. One thing that should be mentioned here is that potentially distracting behaviors can be overcome by using different nonverbal elements. For example, you may find that you naturally cross your arms while talking to others. You can overcome the possible perception that you are acting defensively by using other nonverbal elements, such as smiling, using a friendly tone of voice, or moving closer to the patient. The total message received by the patient is the combination of all nonverbal cues, both positive and negative, and not just one isolated component. Another example is that if you have a soft voice and you sense that the patient cannot hear you, then you can lean toward the patient, raise your voice, or move the patient into a quieter section of the pharmacy. The key to this process is to first recognize distracting nonverbal elements and then try to overcome them.

SUMMARY

Because nonverbal communication contributes significantly to the meanings of messages between pharmacists and patients, it is important for you to keep the following in mind:

1. Certain nonverbal behaviors are universal; yet much of their meanings are based in culture. For example, facial expressions that mean fear, happiness, sadness, or anger may be constant among culturally diverse groups of patients. However, a particular gesture such as a nod of the head may have different meanings in different cultures.

2. Interpreting body language is ambiguous. Many people state that they can read a person like a book. However, some people have been embarrassed by assigning a particular meaning to a specific body movement without checking the meaning of that movement.

3. Nonverbal behavior is more powerful than verbal. If the spoken word contradicts nonverbal behaviors, the observer will believe the nonverbal messages. Even simple advice, such as "Store this in the refrigerator and shake it well every time you use it," may be influenced by your facial expression and tone of voice (Burgoon, et al, 1995). If your tone conveys boredom and your manner is perfunctory, the advice may be seen as being of only minor importance.

4. Your practice environment has an important effect on communication with patients. The location, design elements of the dispensing area, employee appearance, and even the color scheme and signage on the walls all contribute to the messages that patients receive about your philosophy and attitude toward patient counseling.

Nonverbal communication involves an enormously important part of interpersonal communication. You should concentrate on your own nonverbal communications, as well as the various nonverbal cues provided by others. In this way, you can become a more effective, skilled communicator. Developing an awareness of your own nonverbal messages and detecting the nonverbal messages in others are important steps in developing skilled nonverbal communication.

REVIEW QUESTIONS

1. How much communication is attributed to its nonverbal component? Why is this so?
2. What is the importance of cue clusters?
3. List the many ways that body language can improve your role as a pharmacist.
4. Differentiate between kinesics and proxemics.
5. Examine your own nonverbal behavior and list ways you may overcome any distracting styles.

References

Beardsley RS, Johnson CA, Wise G. Privacy as a factor in patient counseling. *Journal of the American Pharmaceutical Association* NS17 (June):366–368, 1977.

Borman EG, Nichols RG, Howell WS, Shapiro GL. *Interpersonal Communication in the Modern Organization.* Englewood Cliffs, NJ: Prentice-Hall, 1969.

Harris L. Physician Patient Barriers to Communication. National Harris Survey, 1997.

Keltner JW. *Interpersonal Communication.* Belmont, CA: Wadsworth, 1970.

McGrath JE, Kelsey JR. *Time and Human Interaction.* New York: Guilford Press, 1989.

Mehrabian A. *Silent Messages.* Belmont, CA: Wadsworth, 1971.

Poytos F. *New Perspectives in Nonverbal Communication.* New York: Pergamon Press, 1983.

Burgoon JK, Buller DB, Woodall WG. *Nonverbal Communication: The Unspoken Dialogue,* 2nd ed. New York: McGraw-Hill, 1995: 251–255.

Chapter 5

Barriers in Communication

▨ OVERVIEW

Within the communication process, numerous barriers exist that could disrupt or even eliminate interpersonal interaction. The potential number of barriers in any pharmacy practice setting is so large that it is a wonder that any communication takes place at all. Interpersonal communication is hindered by environmental barriers, such as crowded, noisy prescription areas; the personal fears and anxieties of both pharmacists and patients; administrative decisions affecting the working environment; and lack of adequate time.

Introduction

Nothing could be more frustrating than to realize that you are not communicating effectively with a person. For example, you want to complain to your car mechanic that your car still does not run right. While you are telling him about your problem, he continues to look at a pile of papers on the counter and to mutter an occasional "uh-huh." You continue to relate in the best way you can the nature and urgency of your problem. However, he rushes over to the phone, papers in hand, and starts talking into the receiver without even looking up. How do you feel—frustrated, angry, confused? Why? Probably because you feel you can't communicate with this person. He is not listening to you.

Although you may never have experienced a situation such as the above, you can probably understand the frustration, anger, and confusion resulting from this lack of communication. Unfortunately, situations in which communication is less than optimal occur frequently.

Removal of communication barriers requires a two-stage process: first, being aware that barriers exist: and, second, taking the appropriate action to overcome them. To become a more effective communicator, it is essential that you realize when you are not communicating effectively with another person and then try to analyze why appropriate communication is not taking place. One or more barriers may be interfering with your communication. This chapter focuses on communication problems and deals with potential barriers to the communication process.

Environmental Barriers

As indicated in Chapter 2, the communication process involves five essential elements: the sender, the message, barriers, the receiver, and feedback. Any of these essential elements may cause a breakdown in communication. The message must be clearly sent and received, and feedback must be related in a clear, unambiguous manner. Distractions in the environment often interfere with this process; therefore, the environment in which communication takes place is critical. Some environmental barriers are rather obvious; others are more subtle.

One of the most obvious barriers is the height of the prescription counter separating the patient from the pharmacist. These prescription counters exist for three primary reasons: (1) they provide an opportunity for patients to identify where the pharmacist is located; (2) they provide the pharmacist with the opportunity to look over the store area periodically; and (3) they provide a private area in which the pharmacist can work. Unfortunately, in some situations patients cannot see the pharmacist behind these strategically placed partitions or counters. It is difficult for patients to talk with pharmacists they cannot even see. This type of environment may give patients the impression that the pharmacist does not want to talk to them. These counters can also intimidate some patients and inhibit communication because the pharmacist is standing over them. Ideally, you and the patient should both be at eye level; this will help counteract perceptions that the pharmacist is not approachable.

Crowded, noisy prescription areas also inhibit one-to-one communication (Beardsley et al, 1977). Many pharmacies tend to have lots of background noise, such as people talking or music playing. These noises interfere with your ability to communicate with the patient. In addition, other people may be within hearing range of your conversation with a patient, which limits the privacy of the interaction. Privacy is especially important when the patient wants to talk about a personal matter. Another subtle barrier is the pharmacist's desire to answer every phone call, which may give the impression that the pharmacist is not willing to talk to the patient.

Privacy does not necessarily mean having a private room, but both the patient and pharmacist must feel that privacy exists. For example, many pharmacists use hanging plants, planters, or dividers to create the feeling of a private conversation area that is away from common traffic areas. Efforts to increase privacy are made fairly easily. For example, many pharmacists use body position (turning away from a busy prescription area) to achieve a more private environment. Paying attention to the amount of privacy can do much to create an atmosphere that causes both pharmacist and patient to communicate with ease.

The presence of a clerk or technician who stands between the patient and pharmacist may be another environmental barrier. In many pharmacies, these assistants are needed to receive and hand prescriptions to patients, handle payments, and help with the over-the-counter purchases. Often, when patients need to talk with the pharmacist, they must first mention it to the clerk, who then relays the message to the pharmacist. In some situations, the pharmacist responds to the assistant (rather than to the patient), who then passes the answer on to the patient. Obviously, this is not the best method of communication, because both the question and answer can be misinterpreted by any of the three parties. Mechanisms that allow patients to have ready access to the pharmacist need to exist.

Ideally, support personnel such as pharmacy technicians do the more technical processing tasks, whereas pharmacists have more contact with patients. Even in work environments in which support staff have initial patient contact, they must be aware of situations in which the patient needs to talk with the pharmacist and must be willing to step aside to allow them to communicate in private. Training your staff in effective communication is a crucial component of your ability to provide appropriate care to patients.

The first step in removing environmental barriers is to find out which ones exist in your practice setting. The best way to do this is to put yourself in the place of the patient (see Box 5.1 for suggested observations). Prescription departments were originally designed to be areas free of traffic so that pharmacists could concentrate on filling prescriptions. Prescription areas were then redesigned so that pharmacists could also watch activity within the pharmacy. Today, demands for meaningful patient–pharmacist dialogue require that the pharmacist be accessi-

---

Box 5.1 POTENTIAL ENVIRONMENTAL BARRIERS

The next time you enter the pharmacy, check for the following:

- Is the pharmacist visible?
- Is it easy to get the pharmacist's attention?
- Does it appear that the pharmacist wants to talk to patients?
- Is the prescription area conducive to private conversation?
- Do you have to speak to the pharmacist through a third party?
- Is there a lot of background noise or other distractions?

---

ble and that an area of privacy be offered. For that to happen, certain physical barriers must be removed so that the pharmacist would need to take as few steps as possible to engage the patient. To accommodate an area for counseling patients, a pharmacy designer should first be consulted to see whether it is possible to make a few simple but effective changes in any traditional prescription area (see Figures 5.1 and 5.2), such as the following:

1. Make countertops wider to accommodate computers and their printer(s).
2. Place a computer terminal near the patient counseling area to minimize the pharmacist's steps.
3. Create a pharmacist–patient interface area that allows easy eye-to-eye contact.
4. Allow a nearby area to be a comfortable waiting area.

Personal Barriers

Many personal characteristics can lead to distractions in communication (Box 5.2). Lack of confidence in personal ability to communicate effectively may influence how people communicate. People who do not believe that they have the ability to communicate well or who are rather shy may avoid talking with others. Many people feel that an effective communication style is something you are born with and may use shyness as an excuse to avoid interacting with others. Unfortunately, people do not realize that communication skills can be learned and developed but, like other skills, require practice and reinforcement. Many times, positive reinforcement for implementing changes in practice may be lacking. A negative experience (e.g., when a pharmacist has had a fight with a customer and realizes that he did not handle the situation well) can be damaging to a person's ego and desire to communicate.

As with most situations, future performance is based on past expe-

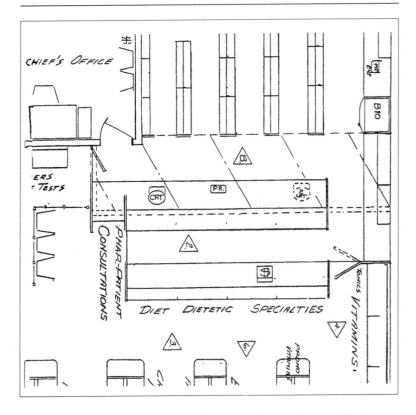

Figure 5.1   A pharmacy designer has created a plan for an effective patient counseling area. (Drawing courtesy of Landon Lovelace Associates, Roanoke, VA)

riences—if you have had good experiences you will be more confident when facing future encounters. You must remind yourself that there are no expert communicators and that no one communicates perfectly 100% of the time. Everyone must strive for an improvement in communication skills by constant practice of new skills.

Another personal barrier is the degree of personal shyness, especially on the part of the pharmacist. Individuals with high levels of shyness tend to avoid interpersonal communication in most situations, including interactions in pharmacy practice settings. These individuals have a high level of anxiety associated with either real or anticipated barriers to communication with others. Overcoming these barriers is a more complex process than overcoming other types of barriers. It requires more time and effort and, many times, professional assistance.

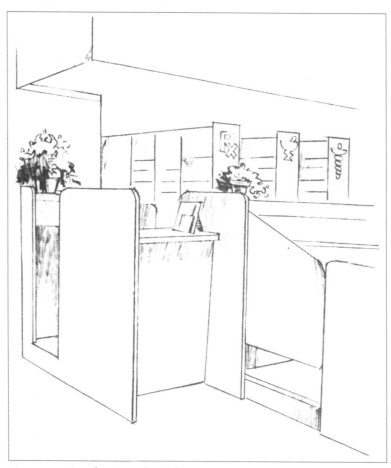

Figure 5.2   By planning ahead for an environment that encourages patients and pharmacists to have face-to-face dialogue, such plans can be translated into a pleasant, efficient, and effective pharmacy area. (Drawing courtesy of Macmillan Healthcare Information)

However, some techniques, such as systematic desensitization or cognitive modification, have been successful for some persons (Baldwin et al, 1982). Since these strategies are far too complex to warrant further discussion in this text, we refer you to counseling psychology literature that discusses these strategies.

Another area that is a personal barrier to communication is the internal conversation you may be having within yourself while talking with others. For example, while you are listening to someone, you may at the same time be arguing within yourself about whether or not you want to deal with this person. This internal conversation or "internal

Box 5.2 EXAMPLES OF PERSONAL BARRIERS

- Low self-confidence
- Shyness
- Dysfunctional internal monologue
- Lack of objectivity
- Cultural differences
- Discomfort in sensitive situations
- Conflicting values to pharmaceutical care practice

monologue" distracts you from listening effectively to another person as you focus your awareness on your own thoughts rather than on what the other person is saying. Often these internal conversations result in your prejudging the person and coming to a hasty conclusion. Internal messages are essential, because they allow you to sort things out while you are communicating, but they can and do become distracting if allowed to take precedence. It is difficult to recognize that you are more preoccupied with your own thoughts than with listening to the other person. It is essential to become aware of this habit because it can inhibit your ability to listen and can make you appear rude.

A further personal barrier involves the tendency of health care providers to take on the emotional problems of patients. Emotional objectivity is important in situations in which you serve many people who have complex problems. As a health care professional, you must attempt to remain empathic but not get so involved that you carry the emotional burden of those with whom you interact. Transferring other people's problems to oneself is emotionally draining—much like losing the charge on a car battery. Eventually, the engine won't start.

Cross-cultural factors, which commonly arise when two people from different cultures interact, may also serve as barriers to effective communication. For example, in some cultures it is not proper to engage in eye contact during communication. From the perspective of these cultures such behavior would be labeled as disrespectful, whereas in others it would be appropriate and almost required. Other cultural factors that may limit communication are (1) different definitions of illness (some patients may not perceive themselves to be ill), (2) different perceptions of what to do when ill (some cultures stress self-reliance rather than seeking help), (3) varying common health-related habits and customs (eating habits), (4) differences in health-seeking behavior (some cultures rely on folk medicine), and (5) perceptions of health care providers (includes possible distrust of the health care system and possible negative past experiences). It is important to recognize that these and other cultural barriers may exist in the patients you serve.

Another personal barrier is the fear of being in a situation that is sensitive or difficult to handle. For example, we may not know exactly what to say when a cancer patient expresses a fear of dying. Or, we may feel awkward when we have to talk to the boss about a sticky personal problem at work. These personal fears or anxieties put tremendous pressure on us to "say the right thing" and may prevent us from talking with others. Often we have blown the situation out of proportion. Once our anxiety about communication is overcome, the situation often turns out better than expected.

Another personal barrier involves a pharmacist's professional values. Many pharmacists believe that talking with patients is not a high-priority activity. They may perceive that patients neither expect nor want to talk with them. It is important to recognize these personal barriers in order to improve interaction. Unlike environmental barriers, removal of these barriers involves personal introspection and analysis of one's motivation and desire to communicate. Removal of these barriers is influenced by pharmacists' ability to change their perceptions. Successful implementation of counseling mandates, such as the Omnibus Budget Reconciliation Act (OBRA) and state regulations, rely on the engagement of pharmacists. If pharmacists do not value patient interaction, then they will not be eager to adopt new patient-centered practices.

Patient Barriers

Several variables relate to patients. For example, patient perceptions of pharmacists are critical in establishing communication rapport. If patients perceive us as not being knowledgeable, they will tend to not ask questions or listen to the advice being offered. Also, if they perceive that we do not want to talk with them, they will not approach us. On the other hand, if patients perceive us as being knowledgeable and have had positive experiences in the past talking with pharmacists, they will tend to seek out information. Therefore, we must alter negative patient perceptions by teaching the patient that we sincerely want to communicate with them and by actually doing so.

Another patient perception that hinders communication is their belief that the health care system is impersonal. Some patients sense that health care providers are not concerned about them as individuals but rather as cases or disease states. They obviously have not been impressed with the empathy displayed by health care providers. You may be seen as a part of this impersonal system. Thus, perception of an impersonal atmosphere may make patients less willing to talk with you or other health care professionals.

Patient perceptions of their medical condition may also inhibit communication. They may believe that their condition is a relatively minor one requiring no further discussion with you or other health care personnel beyond the initial physician visit. In contrast, patients may be anxious about their condition and therefore will avoid talking about it because they feel so vulnerable. In addition, many patients share the perception that if a physician has prescribed a medication, there is no need to know anything more than what is stated on the label. You can convince patients that they need to learn more about their medications, and you can correct some of the patients' inappropriate perceptions about their conditions or medications.

Administrative and Financial Barriers

Several factors dealing with the administrative or financial aspects of pharmacy practice serve as barriers to communication. For example, pharmacists are not paid directly for educating or communicating with patients; therefore, many managers perceive the task of talking with patients as an expensive service and not a high priority. However, studies have shown that many consumers are willing to pay for such service (Smith, 1983; Suh, 2000). In addition, numerous initiatives have begun to document the costs and benefits of patient counseling in an effort to have pharmacists reimbursed by governmental and third-party insurance companies for this valuable service. Community pharmacists are being encouraged by professional organizations to seek reimbursement for the patient care services they provide (Constantine & Scott, 1995; Krinsky, 1999a, 1999b).

Unfortunately, pharmacies have often made policies that discourage pharmacist–patient interaction. Evidence of these policies is reflected in how certain pharmacy practice settings are organized. High prescription counters and glass partitions, or even bars separating patients from the pharmacist, discourage patient–pharmacist interaction. Many pharmacies have limited the number of staff members who can assist pharmacists with their dispensing responsibilities. Shifting the work responsibilities among pharmacy personnel with more pharmacist time freed for direct patient care responsibilities may be necessary to allow pharmacists the chance to counsel patients.

The mechanics of dispensing prescriptions may distract from the communication process. It is difficult to type a label, count medications, talk on the phone, and complete other necessary dispensing tasks while trying to communicate with the patient. The removal of administrative barriers depends on the willingness of management and staff to alter procedures so that patient interaction can be emphasized.

Time Barriers

Choosing an inappropriate time to talk may lead to communication failure. The timing of the interaction is critical, because neither you nor the patient may be ready to communicate at a given time. For example, a woman may have just come from a physician's office where she has waited for three hours with two sick children. The most important thing on her mind is to go home, get her kids to bed, and then relax. She is probably not in the best frame of mind to sit down and have a meaningful conversation with you about the medication. You may also be harried. If a physician is on the phone or a large number of prescriptions need to be filled in a short time, you may feel that this is not a convenient time to talk to the patient. A solution might be to contact the patient by phone or by some other means, such as e-mail, at a later time, when both you and the patient have a more relaxed period in which to communicate. Pharmacists have written information that can reinforce a short message during busy situations. Many pharmacists make efficient use of time by using a variety of strategies, such as "highlighting" a patient information leaflet with a highlight pen to emphasize key points. In any situation, you need to assess nonverbal messages from patients for assurances that communication is well timed (is the patient really listening?).

SUMMARY

Interpersonal communication, because of its complexity and human involvement, is a fragile process. Messages become helpful to the patient only when they are accurately received and understood. If messages are distorted or incorrect, they actually may be harmful to the patient and may prevent a positive patient outcome. Barriers, such as the ones discussed in this chapter, may lead to distortion of messages and misunderstandings between patients and pharmacists. It is important to recognize potential barriers and then to develop a strategy to minimize or remove them.

REVIEW QUESTIONS

1. What is the first step in removing environmental and personal barriers to communication?
2. What are at least three patient barriers that inhibit communication?
3. How can the current nature of pharmacy practice inhibit good communication?

References

Baldwin HJ, Richmond VP, McCroskey JC, Berger BA. Quiet pharmacist. *American Pharmacy* NS22: 24–27, 1982.

Beardsley RS, Johnson CA, Wise G. Privacy as a factor in patient compliance. *Journal of the American Pharmaceutical Association* NS17: 366–368, 1977.

Constantine LM, Scott S. Winning payment for cognitive services: What works. *American Pharmacy* NS35: 14–19, 1995.

Krinsky D. Reimbursement for pharmacist care services. Part 1. *America's Pharmacist* 121: 47–51, 1999a.

Krinsky D. Reimbursement for pharmacist care services. Part 2. *America's Pharmacist* 121: 47–51, 1999b.

Smith D. Willingness of consumers to pay for pharmacists' clinical services. *American Pharmacy* NS23:58–64, 1983.

Suh DC. Consumers' willingness to pay for pharmacy services that reduce risk of medication related problems. *Journal of the American Pharmaceutical Association* 40: 818–827; 876–878, 2000.

Part II
Practical Skills for Pharmacists

art II builds on the essential elements presented in Part I and describes the more complex communication skills needed to provide effective patient care. It addresses the what-, why- and how-type questions involved in the complex skills of listening, assertiveness, interviewing, and assessment. To enhance their skills in these key areas, pharmacists must first become aware of various components of these skills. Next, they must evaluate their performance in each area and, finally, develop strategies to improve their skills in actual practice. Part II focuses on the first step of this process and describes each of these complex skills. Examples of how to identify these skills in a variety of interpersonal situations within pharmacy are also provided. The authors provide guidance in the second and third steps of this process, but readers themselves must perform these assessments in their own personal lives.

Many of the skills discussed in Part II relate to developing better patient care. The collecting and organizing of patient data is built on strong skills discussed in this section. Other complex communication skills could have been included, but the authors chose to focus on the most relevant factors in pharmacy practice. Although most of Part II focuses on pharmacist–patient interaction, these skills are relevant to other types of pharmacist interaction—with other health care providers, employees and employers, and other pharmacists. In other words, interpersonal communication in pharmacy goes beyond patient counseling. Interaction with other individuals by means of the telephone, written mail, electronic mail, or face-to-face must be considered.

Chapter 6

Listening and Empathic Responding

■ OVERVIEW

Listening to patients—trying to understand their thoughts and feelings—is crucial to effective communication. However, empathic communication requires more than understanding. The understanding you have must be conveyed back to patients so they know you understand. In addition, you must genuinely care about patients and not be afraid to communicate your concern to them. Finally, patient feelings must be accepted without judgment as being "right" or "wrong." This chapter examines various skills involved in listening and empathic communication. The attitudes essential to empathic communication and the effects of such communication on pharmacist–patient relationships are also explored.

Listening Well

When we think about skills of "effective communication," we probably think first of the skills involved in speaking clearly and forcefully, that is, in having an effect on others based on what we say. However, an equally critical part of the communication process, and perhaps the most difficult to learn, is the ability to be a good listener. You have probably experienced a sense of satisfaction and gratitude when you have felt that another person really listened to what you had to say and, to a large extent, understood your meaning. In the relationship between the health care professional and the patient, the patient's feeling of being understood is therapeutic in and of itself. It helps to ameliorate the sense of isolation and helplessness that accompanies a patient's experience in negotiating the health care system. Your ability as a pharmacist to provide your patients with this sense of being understood is a crucial part of your effectiveness in communicating with them.

Chapter 2 described the components of the interpersonal communication model and explained the importance of the feedback loop to effective communication. As the receiver of messages, your ability to listen well influences the accuracy with which you are able to decode messages congruent with patients' intended messages. In addition, your ability to convey your understanding back to patients will affect the degree to which they feel understood and cared for. If you fail to understand the patient, this can be uncovered and clarified in the feedback process. If your attempt to listen and understand is genuine, even "missing the mark" will not be damaging if the overall message being conveyed is one of caring and acceptance.

In addition to the communication barriers discussed in previous chapters, some communication habits can interfere with your ability to listen well. Trying to do two things at once makes it evident to patients that they do not have your full attention. Planning what you will say next interferes with your active attempt to understand the meaning of patients' communication. Jumping to conclusions before patients have completed their messages can lead to hearing only parts of messages—often pieces that fit into preconceived ideas that you have. Focusing only on content, judging the person or the message as it is being conveyed, faking interest, communicating in stereotyped ways all cause us to miss much of the meaning in messages that people send us.

Listening well involves understanding both the content of the information being provided and the feelings being conveyed. Skills that are useful in effective listening include (1) summarizing, (2) paraphrasing, and (3) empathic responding. Emphatic responding includes "reflection of feeling" statements that verbally convey your understanding of the essence or emotional meaning of another person's communication. In addition, nonverbal communication that shows caring and attention to the patient is a crucial component of effective listening.

Summarizing

When a patient is providing information, such as during a medication history interview, it is necessary for the pharmacist to try to summarize the critical pieces of information. Summarizing allows you to be sure you accurately understood all that the patient conveyed and allows the patient to add new information that may have been forgotten. Frequent summary statements serve to identify misunderstandings that may exist, especially when there are barriers in communication such as language barriers.

Paraphrasing

When using the technique of paraphrasing, you attempt to convey back to the patient the essence of what he or she has just said. Paraphrasing condenses aspects of content as well as some superficial recognition of the patient's attitudes or feelings. The following are examples of paraphrasing:

PATIENT #1: I don't know about my doctor. One time I go to him and he's as nice as he can be. The next time he's so rude I swear I won't go back again.

PHARMACIST #1: He seems to be very inconsistent.

PATIENT #2: I'm glad I moved into the retirement village. Every day there is something new to do. There are always lots of things going on—I'm never bored.

PHARMACIST #2: So there are a lot of activities to choose from.

EMPATHIC RESPONDING

Empathy Defined

Many of the messages patients send involve the way they feel about their illnesses or life situations. If you are able to communicate back to a patient that you understand these feelings, then a caring, trusting relationship can be established. Communicating that you understand another person's feelings is a powerful way of establishing rapport and is a necessary ingredient in any helping relationship.

Theoretical Foundations

The importance of empathy in helping relationships has been elucidated most eloquently by psychologist Carl Rogers. Rogers developed person-centered psychotherapy, which is part of a humanistic tradition in psychology. Central is the belief that if people are able to express themselves honestly in an accepting, caring atmosphere, they will naturally make healthy, self-actualizing decisions for themselves. In such an environment, people are able to reach solutions to their emotional problems that are right for them. Thus, pharmacists can be helpful by providing a "listening ear" to help patients clarify their feelings. The ability to listen effectively to the emotional meaning in a patient's message is the essence of empathy. Empathy conveys understanding in a caring, accepting, nonjudgmental way. The world is perceived from the patient's point of view. Rogers has noted the lack of empathy in most of our communications (Rogers, 1967):

> I suspect that each of us has discovered that this kind of understanding [empathy] is extremely rare. We neither receive it nor offer it with any great frequency. Instead, we offer another type of understanding, which is very different, such as "I understand what is wrong with you" or "I understand what makes you act that way." These are the types of understanding which we usually offer and receive—an evaluative understanding from the outside. But when someone understands how it feels and seems to me, without wanting to analyze me or judge me, then I can blossom and grow in that climate.

The main difference between an empathic response and a paraphrase is that empathy serves primarily as a reflection of the patient's feelings rather than focusing on the content of the communication. The following examples, adapted from the section on paraphrasing, should illustrate the difference.

PATIENT #1: I don't know about my doctor. One time I go to him and he's as nice as he can be. The next time he's so rude I swear I won't go back again.

PHARMACIST #1: Paraphrase: He seems to be very inconsistent.

EMPATHIC RESPONSE: You must feel uncomfortable going to see him if you never know what to expect from him.

PATIENT #2: I'm glad I moved into the retirement village. Every day there is something new to do. There are always lots of things going on—I'm never bored.

PHARMACIST #2: Paraphrase: So there are a lot of activities to choose from.

EMPATHIC RESPONSE: You seem to love living there.

In addition to using empathic responses, two other attitudes or messages must be conveyed to the patient if trust is to be established. First, you must be genuine, or sincere, in the relationship. If the patient perceives you as phony and your "caring" as a well-practiced facade, then trust will not be established. Being genuine may mean setting limits in the relationship. For instance, it may be necessary to tell a patient that you do not have time right now to discuss an issue in detail, but will telephone or set an appointment when you are not so busy. The fact that you were direct and honest about your limits will probably do less to harm the relationship than if you had said, "I'm listening," while non-verbally conveying hurry or impatience. The incongruence or discrepancy between what we say and how we act sets up barriers that are difficult to overcome.

Another essential condition is respect for and acceptance of the patient as an autonomous, worthwhile person. If you convey an ongoing positive feeling for patients, they may be more open with you, since they do not fear that they are being judged. They are more likely to tell you that they are having trouble taking their medications as prescribed or that they do not understand regimen directions if they know that you will not think them stupid or incompetent. One of the biggest blocks to effective communication is our tendency to judge each other. If we think that another will judge us negatively, we feel less willing to reveal ourselves. Acceptance and warmth, if genuine, allow patients to feel free to be more open in their communication with you.

Empathy and Effective Communication

Empathy has many positive effects. It helps patients come to trust you as someone who cares about their welfare. It also helps them understand their own feelings more clearly. Often their concerns are only vaguely perceived until they begin to talk with someone. In addition, an empathic response facilitates the patient's own problem-solving ability. If they are allowed to express their feelings in a safe atmosphere, patients may begin to feel more in control by understanding their feelings better. Patients may also feel freer to explore possible solutions or different ways of coping with their problems.

As an example, put yourself in the role of a community pharmacist as your patient, Mr. Raymond, talks about his physician: "I've been to Dr. Johnson several times because I heard he was a good doctor. But he just doesn't seem to care. I have to wait endlessly in the waiting room even with an appointment. Then when I do get to see him, he rushes in and out so fast I don't have a chance to talk to him. Oh, he's pleasant enough. I just get the feeling he doesn't have time to talk to me."

Which of the following comes closest to being the type of response you might make to Mr. Raymond? Place a "1" next to a statement that you would definitely use, a "2" next to the statement that you might use, and a "3" next to the statement that you would never use.

_____ a. "You have to understand that Dr. Johnson is a very busy man. He probably doesn't mean to be abrupt."

_____ b. "Dr. Johnson is a very good physician. I'm sure he gives patients the best care possible."

_____ c. "I don't blame you for being upset. You shouldn't have to wait that long when you have an appointment."

_____ d. "Tell him how you feel about the way he treats patients. Otherwise, find a different physician."

_____ e. "I'm sure you just happened to see him when he was having a bad day. I bet if you keep going to him, things will improve."

_____ f. "I know how you feel. I hate to wait in doctors' offices, too."

_____ g. "No one feels that they have enough time to talk with their doctors."

_____ h. "How long do you usually have to wait before you get in to see him?"

_____ i. "Let me talk with you about the new prescription you're getting."

_____ j. "You seem to feel there's something missing in your relationship with Dr. Johnson—that there isn't the caring you would like."

Now that you have indicated which statements appear to be most appropriate, it is important to analyze how Mr. Raymond may perceive each statement. Many times, we attempt to say something that we feel is valuable to patients, but our statements are perceived very differently by the patient. This is due partly to possible hidden messages that we convey. Consider the possible hidden messages that you may have conveyed to Mr. Raymond with each of the above responses.

Judging Response

Although conveying understanding seems so obviously a part of good communication, less helpful types of responses are frequently used in communication with others. Often, for example, we tend to judge or evaluate another's feelings. We tell patients in various ways that they "shouldn't" feel discouraged or frustrated, that they "shouldn't" worry, that they "shouldn't" question their treatment by other health professionals. Any message from you that indicates you think patients are "wrong" or "bad" or that they "shouldn't" feel the way they do will indicate that it is not safe to confide in you. In the previous example, responses (a), "You have to understand that Dr. Johnson is a very busy man. He probably doesn't mean to be abrupt," and (b), "Dr. Johnson is a very good physician. I'm sure he gives patients the best care possible," indicate that you thought Mr. Raymond was "wrong" or that he misperceived the situation. In either case, the judgment was conveyed that he "shouldn't" feel as he does. Even response (c), "I don't blame you for being upset. You shouldn't have to wait that long when you have an appointment," is an evaluative judgment that Mr. Raymond's feelings are "right" and also implies that it is appropriate for you to judge his feelings as "right" or "wrong."

Advising Response

We also tend to give advice. We get so caught up in our role as "expert" or "professional" that we lose sight of the limits of our expertise. We must, as pharmacists, give patients advice on their medication regimens. That is part of our professional responsibility. However, the advising role may not be appropriate in helping a patient deal with emotional or personal problems. The best source of a solution to a problem resides within the patient. It is presumptuous to feel that we can offer a quick solution to another's personal concerns. In addition, it conveys to patients that we do not perceive them as competent to arrive at their own decisions. Even when the advice is reasonable, it is not a decision that patients have arrived at themselves. Relying on others for advice may keep patients dependent, because they see others as the source of problem solving. In the example with Mr. Raymond, your advice in response (d), "Tell him how you feel about the way he treats patients. Otherwise, find a different physician," gives a quick (and rather presumptuous) solution to what is a complex problem in the eyes of Mr. Raymond.

There are times when patients do want advice and are looking for help with their problems. Assisting them in identifying sources of help they can call on may be an appropriate way to help patients. Suggesting alternatives for consideration may also be helpful. In this type of response, you are serving as a sounding board for decisions that the patient makes rather than providing your own solutions.

There are times when patients are not capable of coping with their own feelings or problems. A typical example is the patient who is severely depressed. Being able to recognize the signs of depression and referring patients to sources of help, such as the family physician or a local mental health service, is a professional function you must be prepared to perform. However, most people who are ill have transient feelings of depression and worry that are a normal reaction to the illness. They need to be provided with concerned, empathic care.

Placating or Reassuring Response

A third mode of response to a patient's feelings is a placating or falsely reassuring response. Telling a patient who is facing surgery, "Don't worry, I'm sure your surgery will turn out just fine," may seem to be helpful, but it is really conveying in a subtle way that the person "shouldn't" feel upset. We often use this kind of response to try to get a patient to stop feeling upset or to try to change a patient's feelings rather than accepting the feelings as they exist. This type of response may be used even when the patient is facing a situation of real threat, such as a terminal illness. We may feel helpless in such a situation and use false reassurance to protect ourselves from the emotional involvement of listening and trying to understand the patient's feelings. Response (e), "I'm sure you just happened to see him when he was having a bad day. I bet if you keep going to him, things will improve," is a falsely reassuring response that predicts a positive outcome you have no way of knowing will occur.

Generalizing Response

Another way in which we try to reassure patients is by telling them "I've been through the same thing and I've survived." Although it is comforting to know that others have had similar experiences, this response may take the focus away from the patient experience and onto your own experience before patients have had a chance to talk over their own immediate concerns. It also can lead you to stop listening because you jump to the conclusion that, since you have had an experience similar to the patient's, the patient is feeling the same way you felt. This may not be true. Response (f), "I know how you feel. I hate to wait in doctors' offices, too," would fit in this category. Response (g), "No one feels that they have enough time to talk with their doctors," also indicates that Mr. Raymond's feelings are not unique or special in any way. The "everyone feels that way" response, again, is meant to make Mr. Raymond feel better about his problem but instead makes him feel that you do not consider his concerns to be very unique or important.

Quizzing or Probing Response

Another type of response to feelings is a quizzing or probing response. We feel comfortable asking patients questions—we have learned to do this in medication history taking and in consultations with patients on over-the-counter drugs. However, asking questions when the patient has expressed a feeling can take the focus away from the feeling and onto the "content" of the message. It also leads to the expectation that, if enough information is gathered, a solution will be forthcoming. Many human problems or emotional concerns are not so easily "solved." Often patients simply want to be able to express their feelings and know that we understand. Meeting these needs for a listening ear is an important part of the helping process. Asking Mr. Raymond how long he has to wait for an appointment (response h) does not convey an understanding of the essence of his concern, which was his perception of a lack of caring from his physician.

Distracting Response

Many times we get out of situations to which we don't know how to respond by simply changing the subject. With response (i), "Let me talk with you about the new prescription you're getting," Mr. Raymond gets no indication from you that his concerns have even been heard, let alone understood.

Understanding Response

Contrast each of the other responses to Mr. Raymond with response (j), "You seem to feel there's something missing in your relationship with Dr. Johnson—that there isn't the caring you would like." Only in this response is there any indication that you truly understand the basis of Mr. Raymond's concern. By using such a response, you convey understanding without judging Mr. Raymond as right or wrong, reasonable or unreasonable.

The above discussion reviewed some different responses that you may make to feeling statements. The following dialogue is an example of a patient–pharmacist communication that may invite quite different responses. The situation involves Mrs. Raymond, who engages the pharmacist, Jeff Brown, in conversation when she picks up a prescription for her husband, George. The patient–pharmacist conversation is in the left column, and an analysis of the conversation is in the right column.

Dialogue 1

Conversation

Analysis

Mrs. Raymond: (deep sigh): George has been sick for so long; sometimes I wonder if he's ever going to get well. I don't know if I can keep my spirits up much longer.

Jeff: Now, of course, George is going to get well, and you can keep your spirits up. You've been so strong about it.

Placating response. Mrs. Raymond's reaction to this might be "How can he be so sure George will get well? And he thinks I've been so strong—he has no idea how terrified I've been most of the time."

Conversation	*Analysis*
Mrs. Raymond: But it's been so long. It seems that Dr. Johnson should be getting George well pretty soon.	Mrs. Raymond seems to be protesting Jeff's glib response that she has nothing to worry about.
Jeff: Now, you know Dr. Johnson is a good doctor, and you shouldn't be questioning his care of your husband. It's important to trust your physician.	**Judging response.** Mrs. Raymond's response to this might be "Of course, he'd stick up for the physician. And it isn't really that I question his treatment of George. I'm just frustrated and no one understands that."
Mrs. Raymond: Well, he's certainly not getting anywhere with George!	
Jeff: How long has it been now that George has been sick?	**Quizzing or probing response.** Having this bit of information at this point is probably not as important as focusing on Mrs. Raymond's feelings.
Mrs. Raymond: Thirteen months.	
Jeff: Sometimes these things take time. Maybe you just need to get away more. I think it would do you good to have someone come in and stay with George, say one day a week, so you can get out more.	**Advising response.** While this advice may be reasonable, the fact that Jeff offered this as a quick solution may outrage Mrs. Raymond. It's as if he can presume to tell her how to cope with the situation when she *has* been coping with it for 13 months. If anything, she could probably teach him a thing or two about coping.

Conversation	Analysis
Mrs. Raymond: I don't want to get out more. I want George to get well.	
Jeff: He will, believe me. He is getting the best care possible.	

Contrast the above exchange with the following between Mrs. Raymond and Bill Reynolds, another pharmacist.

Dialogue 2

Conversation	Analysis
Mrs. Raymond (deep sigh): George has been so sick for so long; sometimes I wonder if he's ever going to get well. I don't know if I can keep my spirits up much longer.	
Bill: It must be heartbreaking for you to see George so ill.	**Understanding response.** Bill shows that he recognizes the stress that Mrs. Raymond has been under.
Mrs. Raymond: It is. I sometimes feel that it's hopeless.	Mrs. Raymond confirms that Bill is accurate in his understanding and goes on to reveal a little more about her feelings.
Bill: You seem discouraged.	
Mrs. Raymond (head nod and nonverbal struggle to control tears)	Often the response to an accurate understanding will not be further exploration of feelings. The fact that someone has listened and understood may be all she needs at the time. Bill lets her decide how much she wishes to reveal by leaving the door open without forcing disclosure through probing.
Bill (after long pause): Is there something I can do to help?	

Conversation	*Analysis*
Mrs. Raymond: Sometimes it helps just to be able to talk to people. Dr. Johnson always tells me not to worry. How can I help but worry?	
Bill: It sounds as if people try to cheer you up instead of understanding how difficult it is for you.	
Mrs. Raymond: I don't blame Dr. Johnson. I know he's a good doctor. But sometimes I get frustrated by how long it's taking.	

A patient who feels discouraged or angry often needs simply to know that others understand. Mrs. Raymond is not "blaming" Bill or the physician but is lashing out because of her own frustrations and feelings of helplessness. Rather than placating her or judging her feelings (you shouldn't let yourself get discouraged), the pharmacist can be helpful by showing concern and understanding.

We try in various ways to get patients to stop or change their feelings. We may feel uncomfortable in dealing with expressions of emotion; so, to protect ourselves we cut off patients' communication of feelings. We may try to distract them by changing the subject; we may try to show them that things are not as bad as they seem; or, we may direct the communication to subjects we feel comfortable with, such as medication regimens. These responses tend to convey to patients that we are not listening and perhaps that we do not *want* to listen. It is a gratifying experience for patients to feel that someone has listened and, to a large extent, understands their feelings. As a pharmacist, monitoring how well you are listening to patients is as important as carefully choosing the words you use in educating them about their medications.

Attitudes Underlying Empathy

Underlying empathic responding is an empathic attitude toward others. This attitude means that you want to listen and try to understand people's feelings and points of view. It means you are able to accept feelings as they exist without trying to change them, stop them, or judge them. You are not afraid of a patient's emotions and are able to just *be* with the person and not necessarily *do* anything except listen. An empathic person is able to trust that people can cope with their own feelings and problems. If this attitude is held, you will not be afraid to allow patients to express their feelings and arrive at their own decisions. An empathic person also believes that listening to someone is helpful in itself and is often the only means of help one has to offer.

Health professionals feel frustrated when they cannot prescribe a medication and "cure" a patient's problems. Yet, the emotional concerns that patients bring along with their physical problems cannot be cured or treated in that way. This does not mean that you have no help to provide; it does mean that you must define "helping" in a new way.

In empathic communication, it is not sufficient to feel that you understand another person—empathy requires that you effectively convey to the person that you do really understand. How can this be done? One approach is to briefly summarize or capsulize what you understand the person's feelings to be. In the conversation between the second pharmacist (Bill) and Mrs. Raymond, Bill said "You seem discouraged," which captured the essence of what Mrs. Raymond had been communicating and served to convey to her that Bill had heard and understood her concerns.

The ability to capsulize the essence of a patient's feelings and convey this understanding back to the patient often involves what is called "reflection of feeling." Reflection of feeling has been defined as restating in your own words the essential attitudes and feelings expressed by the patient. Reflection of feeling is not simply a repetition of what the patient has said; instead, it conveys your attempt to grasp the meaning of the patient's communication. It further implies that you are checking to make sure that your understanding is accurate. In this sense, the reflection of feeling is not a bold, declarative statement but is tentative and provisional. For example, Mrs. Raymond describes another problem to Judy Lang, the pharmacist:

> My daughter seems to get sick a lot—headaches or nausea and vomiting. I've had her to the doctor, but he says there's nothing wrong. I've noticed that she seems to get sick whenever there's a big exam she's supposed to take or a speech she's supposed to give at school. It isn't that I think she's faking, mind you. She really is sick—vomiting and everything.

If Judy were to respond "Your daughter seems to get sick a lot—usually right before a big exam at school," she is simply repeating what Mrs. Raymond has told her. Mrs. Raymond might reasonably respond, "That's what I just told you, isn't it?" However, if Judy were to go beyond the surface meaning of Mrs. Raymond's statement and try to reflect her concern in fresh words, Judy's response might be something like this: "It sounds as if you're afraid your daughter may be reacting to the stress she feels at school by becoming physically ill. Is that what you think is happening?"

Judy's response captured Mrs. Raymond's concern but was put into Judy's own words and so was perceived by Mrs. Raymond as showing understanding. In this response, Judy did not jump to unreasonable or unsupported conclusions about what the problem was. Her response is a tentative "let's see if I understand" kind of response. In addition, she avoided any threatening labels or interpretations such as "You seem to feel your daughter's illnesses are psychosomatic." Such a word would have been too "clinical" and frightening for Mrs. Raymond and would have hindered Judy's attempt to show understanding.

If Judy had tried to convey her understanding by saying "I know how you feel" or "I understand your concern," the response would not have been as effective as a reflection of feeling response in conveying empathy. "I understand" is a cliché that can be used as a standard response to any feeling statement and thus is not perceived as a response unique to the person with whom you are talking. Because the response also does nothing to convey what your understanding is, it is much less personal and effective than actually trying to reflect the feeling the person is expressing.

An empathic response implies neither agreement nor disagreement with the perceptions of the patient. If a patient says to you as manager of a pharmacy, "Your clerk was extremely rude to me. She acts as if she doesn't care about your customers," your first impulse may be to check the facts. This is important and necessary, but it does not convey understanding of the patient's perceptions. The patient talking to you does not *feel* cared for, regardless of what the objective truth about the clerk's behavior happens to be.

Empathy *Can* Be Learned

There is a widespread belief that empathic communication skills are not something one can learn. The belief is based on the notion that you either are an empathic person or you are not. As with any new behavior, learning to alter existing habits of responding *is* very difficult. Pharmacists who are not accustomed to conveying their understanding of the meaning of illness and treatment for their patients will at first feel awkward using empathic responses. As with any new skill, being an empathic listener must be practiced before it can become a natural part of how we relate to others. However, empathic communication skills can be learned if people have value systems that place importance on establishing therapeutic relationships with patients. As health care providers, we must develop a certain level of caring for patients and learn how to be better listeners.

Empathy and Trust in Health Professional–Patient Relationships

The trust that patients have in their health care providers means that they have confidence that providers will act in their best interests. Mechanic and Meyer (2000) describe the vulnerability of patients and the risks they take in trusting people they hardly know (health professionals) in circumstances in which misplaced trust can have devastating consequences. These investigators identified **interpersonal** (not technical) competence as the principal component mentioned by patients as key to trust in their providers. The traits identified most often were provider willingness to listen and their ability to display caring, concern, and compassion. In addition to helping establish trust in patient–provider relationships, provider recognition of appropriate response to patient emotional distress has been found to be related to actual reduction in patient emotional distress (Roter et al, 1995).

Nonverbal Aspects of Listening

In conveying your willingness to listen, your nonverbal behavior is at least as important as what you say. You can do a number of things nonverbally to convey your interest and concern. Establishing eye contact while talking to patients, leaning toward them with no physical barriers between you, and having a relaxed posture all help to put the patient at ease and show your concern. Head nods and encouragements to talk are also part of empathic communication. A tone of voice that conveys that you are trying to understand the person's feelings also complements the verbal message. Establishing a sense of privacy by coming out from behind the counter and getting away from others who may be waiting helps convey your respect for the patient. Conveying that you have time to listen—that you aren't hurried or distracted—makes your concern seem genuine.

Sensitivity to the nonverbal cues of patients is also a necessary part of effective communication. Asking yourself, "how is this person feeling?" during the course of a conversation will lead to the discovery that feelings and attitudes are often conveyed most dramatically (sometimes exclusively) through nonverbal channels. A person's tone of voice, facial expression, and body posture all convey messages about feelings. To be empathic, you must "hear" these messages as well as the words patients use.

Problems in Establishing Helping Relationships

There are countless sources of problems in interpersonal communication between pharmacists and patients. However, certain pharmacist attitudes and behaviors are particularly damaging in establishing helping relationships with patients. These include stereotyping, depersonalizing, and controlling behaviors. The following section describes these common deficiencies and offers suggestions for improvement in these key areas.

Stereotyping

Communication problems may exist because of negative stereotypes held by health care practitioners that affect the quality of their communication. What image comes to mind when you think of an elderly patient...welfare patient...an AIDS patient...a chronic pain patient...a noncompliant patient...an illiterate patient...a hypochondriacal patient...a dying patient...a psychiatric patient? Even the label "patient" may create artificial or false expectations of how any individual might behave.

If you hold certain stereotypes of patients, you may fail to listen without judgment. In addition, information that confirms the stereotype may be perceived while information that fails to confirm it is *not* perceived. For example, if a pharmacist has a negative stereotype of people who use analgesics, especially opioids, on a long-term basis, he or she may view a patient who complains about lack of effective pain control as "drug seeking" rather than as someone who is not receiving appropriate therapy.

What does the issue of stereotyping mean for pharmacists? First, before we can be effective in communicating with patients, we must come to know what stereotypes we hold and how these may affect the care we give our patients. We must then begin to see our patients as individuals with the vast array of individual differences that exist. Only then can we begin to relate to each patient as a person, unique and distinct from all others.

Depersonalizing

Unfortunately, there are a number of ways in which communication with a patient can become depersonalized. If an elderly person is accompanied by an adult child, for example, we may direct the communication to the child and talk about the patient rather than with the patient. We may also focus communication on "problems" and "cases." Many aspects of disease management make communication narrow and impersonal. For example, discussing only the disease or the problems a patient might have managing treatment without commenting on the successes in treatment or even the everyday aspects of the patient's life places the focus on narrow clinical rather than broader personal issues. A rigid communication format of a pharmacist monologue rather than pharmacist–patient dialogue can also make communication seem rote and defeat the underlying purpose of the encounter.

Controlling

Numerous studies have found that an individual's sense of control is related to health and feelings of well-being (Rodin, 1986; Langer, 1983; Taylor et al, 2000). A review of literature (Taylor et al, 2000) concluded that beliefs such as perceived personal control and optimism actually protect both the mental and physical health of individuals. When health care providers do things that reduce the patient's sense of control over decisions that are made regarding treatment, they may actually be reducing the effectiveness of the therapies they prescribe.

Fostering a sense of control in patients is important in patient–practitioner relationships (see Schorr and Rodin, 1982, for a description of the theoretical foundation). Interventions to increase levels of patient participation and control in the provider–patient relationship have yielded positive results that include improved clinical and quality of life outcomes (Kaplan et al, 1989). Still, actual communication between health care providers and patients may decrease rather than enhance the perceived personal control of the patient (Schorr and Rodin, 1982). Illness often results in disturbing feelings of helplessness and dependence on health care providers. Added to this patient vulnerability is the unequal power in relationships between providers and patients and the tendency of providers to all too often adopt an authoritarian style of communicating. Patients are "told" what they should do and what they should not do. Decisions are made, often with very little input from the patient regarding their preferences, desires, or concerns about treatment.

Nevertheless, in the process of carrying out treatment plans, patients do make decisions about their regimens—decisions that we may remain unaware of. In this way, patients reassert control of the management of their own conditions. Labeling certain patient decisions as "noncompliance" is not helpful. Such labeling misses the point that the goal of treatment is to help patients improve health and well-being; it is *not* to get them to do as they are told. Rather than blaming the patient, we must appreciate the degree to which treatment decisions are inevitably shared decisions. We must ensure that information and feedback are conveyed by both patients and ourselves in a give-and-take process. We must actively encourage patients to ask questions and urge them to discuss problems they perceive with treatment, to discuss complaints they have about their therapy, or to discuss frustrations they feel concerning their progress. This encouragement requires above all else our empathic acceptance of the patient's feelings and perceptions. Patient input is not seen as peripheral to the provision of health care. Instead, we see the patient as the center of the healing process. Establishing a relationship in which patients are active participants in making treatment decisions and in assessing treatment effects is crucial to provision of quality care.

SUMMARY

Listening well is not a passive process; it takes involvement and effort. It also takes practice to convey understanding in a way that seems natural rather than mechanical or artificial. However, when a relationship between you and a patient is marked by empathic understanding, the patient is helped in ways medications cannot touch.

REVIEW QUESTIONS

1. Describe each of the four skills of effective listening: summarizing, paraphrasing, empathic responding, and nonverbal attending.
2. Empathic responding has several positive effects. What are they?
3. How can active listening be inhibited by stereotyping, depersonalizing, and controlling.

References

Kaplan SH, Greenfield S, Ware JE, Jr. Assessing the effects of physician-patient interactions on the outcomes of chronic disease. *Medical Care* 27:5110–5127, 1989.

Langer EJ. *The Psychology of Control.* Beverly Hills, CA: Sage, 1983.

Mechanic D, Meyer S. Concepts of trust among patients with serious illness. *Social Science and Medicine* 51:657–668, 2000.

Rodin J. Aging and health: effects of the sense of control. *Science* 233:1271–1276, 1986.

Rogers CB. The therapeutic relationship: recent theory and research. In Patterson CH, ed. *The Counselor in the School.* New York: McGraw-Hill, 1967.

Roter DL, Hall JA, Kern DE, et al. Improving physicians' interviewing skills and reducing patients' emotional distress: a randomized clinical trial. *Archives of Internal Medicine* 155:1877–1884, 1995.

Schorr D, Rodin J. The role of perceived control in practitioner-patient relationships. In Wills TA, ed. *Basic Processes in Helping Relationships.* New York: Academic Press, 1982.

Taylor SE, Kemeny ME, Reed GM, et al. Psychological resources, positive illusions, and health. *American Psychologist* 55:99–109, 2000.

Recommended Readings

Barnard D, Barr JT, Schumacher GE. Empathy. In The American Association of Colleges of Pharmacy: Eli Lilly Pharmacy Communication Skills Project. Bethesda, MD: AACP, 1982.

Bernstein L, and Bernstein RS. *Interviewing: A Guide for Health Professionals,* 4th ed. Norwalk, CT: Appleton-Century-Crofts, 1985.

Chapter 7

Assertiveness

▨ OVERVIEW

Assertive pharmacists take an active role in patient care. These pharmacists initiate communication with patients rather than wait to be asked questions. Assertive pharmacists also convey their views on the management of patient drug therapy to other health care professionals. Finally, assertive pharmacists try to resolve conflicts with others in a direct manner but in a way that conveys respect for others.

Beginning Exercise

Before reading further, stop and ask yourself these questions:

1. If a group in your community asks you to give a speech on medication use, how would you respond?
2. When a patient is hostile, how do you tend to respond?
3. How many patients and physicians you talk with know you by name?
4. How often do you make it a point to talk with patients who are getting new prescriptions to make sure they understand their

therapy? How often do you counsel only when they ask questions?

5. How frequently do you look at profile records and ask patients questions during refill visits to make sure medications are being taken appropriately, that therapeutic goals are being met, and that there are no problems with therapy?

The questions posed may seem to deal with diverse, unrelated situations—giving speeches, coping with criticism, and counseling patients. Yet they all involve situations in which you can choose to act assertively or nonassertively.

Defining Assertiveness

What is assertiveness? Assertiveness is perhaps best understood by comparing it with two other response styles: passivity and aggression. These three styles of responding are described in the following text.

Passive Behavior

The passive response is designed to avoid conflict at all cost. Passive or nonassertive persons do not say what they really think out of fear that others may not agree. Passive individuals "hide" from people and wait for others to initiate conversation. They put others' needs or wants above their own. Problems arise when people who behave passively feel secretly angry or resentful toward others. Passive persons may see themselves as victims who are subject to the manipulation of others. This view is damaging to their self-esteem.

Aggressive Behavior

Aggressive people seek to "win" in conflict situations by dominating or intimidating others. Aggressive persons promote their own interests or points of view but are indifferent or hostile to the feelings, thoughts, and needs of others. Often, aggression seems to work because others back down to avoid prolonging or escalating the conflict. However, persons who give in to the intimidation of aggressive individuals may also act in subtle ways to "get even." For example, patients who do not feel they are treated with respect in a community pharmacy may not return to that pharmacy and may tell friends about their negative experiences. Employees who feel helpless can sabotage the goals of their employer in a variety of indirect ways. Thus, aggressive persons may "win" certain arguments in the short term, but their behavior may lead to negative long-term consequences.

Assertive Behavior

Assertive behavior is the direct expression of ideas, opinions, and desires. The intent of assertive behavior is to communicate in an atmosphere of trust. Conflicts that arise are faced and solutions of mutual accord are sought. Assertive individuals initiate communication in a way that conveys their concern and respect for others. The goal of communication is to stand up for oneself and to solve interpersonal problems in ways that do not damage relationships with others. Assertiveness implies that you respect the rights of others and also value your own beliefs and opinions.

The critical factor in being assertive is the ability to act in ways that are consistent with the standards we have for our own behavior. When we tell ourselves that other people "make" us feel or act a certain way, we are not taking responsibility for our own behavior. Instead of changing ourselves, we try (impotently) to get others to change. We believe that, as Mark Twain noted, "nothing so needs reform as other people's habits." However, the only power we have to effect change in any relationship is to change our own behavior. For example, you may wish that your boss, who tends to be very negative during annual performance evaluations of staff, were more supportive of your work. However, just hoping that she would be more positive in her evaluations will not resolve this issue. You must take active steps to change how you respond to her criticisms rather than wait for her to change her approach.

Too often, our goals in communication are defined in terms of what we want others to do rather than what *we* will do. For example, we might say that we want physicians to appreciate the role of the pharmacist in patient care. Redefining this goal would have us focus on what specific things we can do to improve our working relationships with physicians. If we tell others our goals in providing pharmaceutical care services and show them by our behavior what we want to achieve, many will come to respect our position. However, even if we fail to convince a physician that the role we play in patient care is of value, it does not mean that we have failed in reaching the goals we have set for our own communication. When our goals focus on what we will do, we have control over our ability to meet these goals.

Research has shown that a number of skills are needed for assertive communication. These include initiating and maintaining conversations, encouraging assertiveness in others, responding appropriately to criticism, giving negative feedback acceptably, expressing appreciation or pleasure, making requests, setting limits or refusing requests, conveying confidence both verbally and nonverbally, and expressing opinions and feelings appropriately. Several of these strategies are described in a section on assertive techniques later in this chapter.

Theoretical Foundations

Assertiveness training and theories about how people learn to respond in passive or aggressive ways grow primarily out of cognitive and behaviorist psychological theories. Behaviorists believe that passive or aggressive responses have been reinforced or rewarded and thus strengthened. Aggressive behavior often works in the short term because others feel intimidated and allow aggressive persons to get what they want. Passive behaviors are reinforced when individuals are able to escape or even avoid conflict in relationships and thus escape the anxiety that surrounds these conflicts.

Cognitive theories hold that people respond passively or aggressively because they hold irrational beliefs that interfere with assertiveness. These beliefs involve:

1. Fear of rejection or anger from others and need for approval (everyone should like me and approve of what I do)
2. Overconcern for the needs and rights of others (I should always try to help others and be nice to them)
3. Belief that problems with assertiveness are due to unalterable personality characteristics and are therefore unchangeable (this is just how I am)
4. Negative self-evaluation combined with perfectionist standards (I must be perfectly competent. If I am not, then I am a failure)

Because these beliefs are excessively perfectionistic, they are considered irrational. In the nonassertive person, they create anxiety that leads the individual to try (unsuccessfully) to avoid the inevitable conflicts that arise in relationships. These unrealistic standards are also turned on others, leading to angry, aggressive behavior, with frequent "blaming" of others for normal human failings. *Cognitive restructuring*, an assertiveness technique, teaches people to identify self-defeating thoughts that produce anxiety or inappropriate anger in difficult situations and replace them with more reasonable thoughts. As these new thoughts replace the self-defeating thoughts, they begin to be incorporated into the person's belief system. For example, as a pharmacist you may feel "used" by a boss who always counts on you for emergency coverage. You might currently say to yourself "I don't want to come to work on my day off this week, but if I say 'no' the boss will get mad and that would be awful." Because this causes you anxiety at the imagined catastrophic consequences of saying "no," your response is inhibited. A more rational thought process when faced with such a request would be "I don't want to work on my day off this week. It is my right to say no. I am not responsible for solving all the problems my manager has in finding back-up coverage." This thought reduces anxiety and frees you to practice new, more assertive responses to difficult situations.

Assertiveness Techniques

There are a number of communication techniques or strategies that are useful in responding to situations that tend to be conflict-ridden.

Providing Feedback

Letting others know how you respond to their behavior can help to prevent misunderstandings and also help to resolve the conflicts that are inevitable in relationships. However, providing honest feedback when you have a negative reaction to another person's behavior is difficult to accomplish without hurt feelings. Many times, you must tell people you are upset by what they did in order to improve your relationship in the long run. One strategy is to use effective feedback to make the communication less threatening. The following are criteria for useful feedback:

- Feedback focuses on a person's behavior rather than personality. By focusing on behavior, you are directing the feedback to something the individual can change.
- Feedback is descriptive rather than evaluative. Describing what was said or done is less threatening than judging why you assume it was done.
- Feedback focuses on your own reactions rather than the other person's intentions. Assigning "blame" or assuming malevolent intent behind the behavior is not part of constructive feedback.
- Feedback is specific rather than general. It focuses on behavior that has just occurred and avoids dragging in past behavior. It also does not overgeneralize from the specific instance that has upset you (e.g., "you always do ___").
- Feedback focuses on problem solving. The intent is **not** to let off steam. The intent is to solve a problem in a relationship so that the relationship can be improved.
- Feedback is provided in a private setting.

Inviting Feedback from Others

We need to work on providing feedback in an appropriate manner. At the same time, we need to invite feedback from others to improve our interpersonal communication skills. For example, as a pharmacist, you should routinely assess patient satisfaction and invite feedback on your services. As a manager, you should let employees know that you welcome suggestions from them on how to improve pharmacy operations. Your ability to hear criticism or suggestions without defensiveness or anger, to admit when you have made a mistake, and to encourage feedback from others (even when it is negative) encourages people to be honest in their communications with you. It also allows you to identify areas of your professional practice that may need improvement and promotes better relationships with others.

Setting Limits

For some of us, setting limits on how we spend our personal time and money is a source of frustration. We have difficulty saying "no" to any request. As a result, we feel overwhelmed and often angry at others for "taking advantage" of us. Being assertive in limit setting means taking responsibility for the decisions on how to spend personal resources without feeling resentful toward others for making requests. Being assertive in limit setting does not mean that you stop saying "yes" to requests. You will no doubt continue to help others, even though doing so may be an inconvenience, because of the value system you hold and your desire to help others when they need help.

When faced with a request, the first step is to decide how much you are willing to do in meeting that request. If you need time to decide, delaying a response is appropriate as long as you get back to the person within the time frame you specify. Often, a response may not be yes or no but an offer to partially meet the request. Saying no or setting limits may be particularly difficult if you believe that the other person must agree that you have a good reason for saying no. If feelings of guilt trap you, you may not want to provide specific reasons for your decisions. Whether you give reasons or not does not change the fact that you have the right to make the decision on how you spend personal time and financial resources.

Making Requests

Asking for what you want from others in a direct manner is also necessary in healthy relationships. If you are in a management position, clearly communicating your expectations of others is an important part of carrying out the goals of the organization. In equal relationships, making requests, including asking for help, is an important part of honest communication. We must trust that others will be able to respond to our requests in an assertive manner, including saying no. Thus, we must not overreact when someone turns down our request in an assertive way.

Being Persistent

One important aspect of being assertive is to be persistent in ensuring that your rights are respected. Often, when you have set limits or say no, people try to coax you into changing your mind. If you continue to repeat your decision calmly, you can be assertive without becoming aggressive and without giving in. This response of calmly repeating your decision is often called the "broken record" response (Smith, 1975). It will stop even the most manipulative person without assigning blame or escalating the conflict.

Ignoring Provocations

Interpersonal conflict may elicit various ways of trying to "win" by attempting to humiliate or intimidate others. For example, patients who are angry or feeling helpless may lash out with personal attacks. Pharmacists who feel unfairly criticized may respond in an aggressive or sarcastic manner. Interpersonal conflicts between health professionals are often marked by struggles for power and autonomy (often called "turf battles"). Ignoring the critical comments of others and focusing exclusively on solving underlying problems can do much to keep conflict from escalating to the point that relationships are damaged.

Responding to Criticism

For some of us, criticism is particularly devastating because we typically hold two common irrational beliefs: (1) that we must be loved or approved of by others and (2) that we must be completely competent in everything we do and never make mistakes. Since such perfectionist standards are impossible to achieve, we are constantly faced with feelings of failure or unworthiness. In some cases, we may even have a desire to "get even" by launching into a counterattack on the person levying the criticism. The only way to counteract such feelings—and to begin to cope reasonably with criticism—is to begin to challenge the underlying, irrational beliefs that lead us to fear the disapproval of others.

How do assertiveness problems relate to your ability to function more effectively as a pharmacist? Let's examine a few typical situations in pharmacy practice and determine what might be the most assertive way to respond in relationships with patients, physicians, employees, employers, and colleagues.

Assertiveness and Patients

Perhaps the most important assertiveness skill in relating to patients is your willingness to initiate communication. Certain activities distinguish assertive pharmacists from passive ones. For example, some pharmacists seem to hide behind the counter, give prescriptions to clerks to hand to patients, and generally avoid interaction with patients unless asked specific questions. In this way, passive pharmacists are able to avoid the potential conflicts inherent in dealing with people and are able to hide their own feelings of insecurity and fears about being incompetent. Although a passive approach may arise out of (or at least be rationalized by) a feeling of time pressure, passive pharmacists make no attempt to find alternative ways of providing better patient care, such as giving patients well-developed medication leaflets and calling them during slower hours to discuss key points and assess problems. Instead, passive pharmacists deal with things as they come and take the path of least resistance in providing minimal levels of pharmacy services. Assertive pharmacists come out from behind counters, introduce themselves to patients, provide information on medications, and assess the patient's use of medications and problems with therapy.

Encouraging patients to be more assertive is also an important skill in improving your communication with patients. Helping patients prepare for visits with health professionals and encouraging their active participation in consultations has been found to improve communication and make patients more assertive in asking questions (Kaplan et al, 1989; Kimberlin et al, 2001; Roter, 1977, 1984). As a pharmacist, you may encourage patients to be more assertive by suggesting that they keep a list of questions that they want to ask about their therapy during their next visit. You may also have patients fill out brief questionnaires when they arrive at the pharmacy on which they write down their questions or concerns about their health or treatment. You could even give them a short checklist of informational items or issues about medications and ask them to check the items they would like to discuss with you. This process can help patients organize their thoughts and can counteract the passivity that patients may adopt in the presence of a health professional. During their visits, you can actively solicit questions, concerns, and preferences regarding health care. Even normally assertive patients may experience enough anxiety in communication with providers that they forget to ask questions or bring up concerns they have.

REVIEW CASE 7.1

A patient who is obviously in a hurry brings in a prescription to be filled. You are extremely busy, and there is a 30-minute wait. When she is told this, she explodes "That is ridiculous. It can't take that long to pour pills from a big bottle into a little bottle." When you start to explain about patient counseling, she says "I've never had anyone talk with me about the prescriptions I get here. All you do is ask me to sign a form."

What special assertiveness skills might you use?

What is your role in this situation?

A particularly difficult situation that you will face in pharmacy practice is responding to an angry or critical patient. No one likes to hear criticism, but there are ways of dealing with criticism in a rational, assertive manner. When you hear criticism from patients (such as in Case 7.1), it is important to keep in mind that their feelings of hostility may be greatly magnified by the life stresses they are experiencing. Patients are usually ill, sometimes seriously ill, and may be feeling helpless and dependent on health professionals. They may feel shuffled about, kept waiting in physician offices, and finally kept waiting for a prescription. It is important, therefore, to keep in mind that some (do not assume "all") patient anger arises from frustrations about being ill and not from personal grievances against you.

When patients are reacting primarily to the stresses of being ill, it is most helpful to understand what it is like for them and to respond empathically. An empathic response when patients react with shock and dismay at the cost of their medications is probably more helpful than an attempt to justify the cost. Saying, "You're right. These medications are expensive. Are you worried about whether you can afford them?" shows that you understand the patient's worry and allows you to assess whether the concern about cost is a real problem of inability to afford treatment or a way of expressing diverse feelings of frustration.

Another skill that is useful in responding to patient criticism is to get patients to turn criticism into useful feedback. For example, if a patient tells you that your pharmacy does not seem to care about the customer, it is important to find out specifically what is causing the problem. Ask: "What specifically is it that upsets you?" This may give you feedback that would be useful in improving your pharmacy operation. You now have the information that you need to decide whether you should make changes to improve patient care. Alternatively, you may decide to continue with current policies, but see the need to better communicate your reasons for these decisions to patients.

Assertiveness and Physicians

When problems in patient medication therapies arise, consultations with physicians are often required. If you have determined that you need to speak directly with the physician, persistence with receptionists and nurses in your request will be most effective. Messages transmitted through third parties may not be the most effective means of communication. Such persistence might sound something like this:

PHARMACIST (TO PHYSICIAN'S NURSE): This is John Landers, the pharmacist at Central Pharmacy, I'd like to speak to Dr. Stone, please.

NURSE: He's with a patient right now. What is it you wish to speak to him about?

PHARMACIST: I am concerned about Mrs. Raymond's prescription for metformin. I will need to speak to Dr. Stone about it. Please have him call me as soon as he comes out from the patient examination.

NURSE: It might be quicker if you tell me what the problem is. I could talk to Dr. Stone and get back to you.

PHARMACIST: Thank you, but in this case I would like to talk to Dr. Stone directly.

NURSE: He's very busy today and we're running behind schedule.

PHARMACIST: I know he has a busy schedule, but I must speak with him as soon as possible. Please ask him to call.

The pharmacist in this communication was assertive. He showed respect for the nurse and yet was persistent in stating his request. He did not argue about the issue of which method of communication was quicker. He calmly restated his request without anger or apology.

Now, let's say you have managed to get through to the physician. Compare the following introductory comments by a pharmacist.

a. Dr. Stone, this is the pharmacist at Main Street Pharmacy. I'm sorry to bother you—I know you're busy—but I think there's a problem with Mrs. Raymond's prescription for metformin.

b. Dr. Stone, this is John Landers, the pharmacist at Main Street Pharmacy. I'm calling about a problem Mrs. Raymond is having with her prescription for metformin.

In (a), the pharmacist did not introduce himself, which makes him an anonymous employee of a pharmacy rather than a professional with an individual identity. Also, in (a), he subtly "apologizes" for calling, which makes him seem insecure and unassertive.

Here are several ways the pharmacist could precede:

a. Did you know that Mrs. Raymond is still having diarrhea from the metformin? Do you want to change her prescription?

b. I spoke with Mrs. Raymond today. She reports that she continues to have diarrhea after 3 months on the medication. She has stopped her walking program and is reluctant to leave the house because of the diarrhea. The effect on her life is so serious that you may want to consider switching her to a sulfonylurea such as glyburide or one of the newer thiazolidinediones such as Avandia (rosiglitazone) or Actos (pioglitazone), which are less likely to cause diarrhea.

Response (b) is better. The pharmacist is not putting the physician on the spot by asking him if he knew there was a problem. Rather, he presented the problem that concerned him and suggested alternative medications that could possibly resolve the problem.

When identifying potential problems, be prepared to identify alternatives to try to resolve the problem and to make your own recommendation on the preferred alternative. To do this with confidence, you should have checked references before making the phone call or sending the written communication. Having information on current research and citing it to convince the physician will increase your effectiveness in making a recommendation. Once you are sure of your facts, it is easier to be persistent in pushing for a therapeutic change that is required. Be sure that you feel prepared to use the medical terms and speak to the physician as a fellow health professional. Focus on the goal you share with the physician, which is to help the patient. When changes in therapy are agreed to, it should be clear how the changes will be implemented (e.g., who will inform the patient) and what the monitoring plan will be to verify that the patient's problem has been resolved.

You are faced with many barriers to communicating effectively with physicians. Physicians may not accept recommendations and may actually seem ungrateful to some of your interventions. Even when you do effect a change in physician behavior, you may not receive feedback that your efforts have been successful. Perhaps the next prescription the physician writes will show a change, even though the physician's initial response to you indicated that a change would not be made. Unfortunately, you are not always going to get a "pat on the back" for consultations with physicians.

It is important to keep in mind, therefore, that consulting with physicians when problems arise or asking questions when something seems to be a problem must be done in spite of what the physician's reaction might be. To fail to consult a physician because of anticipated resistance reduces your professional role to one of subservience—one in which you are willing to abdicate your responsibilities as a health professional or fail to act in the patient's best interest because you feel uncomfortable carrying out these patient care functions.

Although pharmacists seem to fear that physicians will not respond positively to therapeutic recommendations, the research evidence suggests just the opposite. Research from a number of different pharmacy practice environments indicates that, when pharmacists make suggestions to physicians for important therapeutic changes in a patient's drug treatment, in the vast majority of cases, pharmacist recommendations are accepted and implemented by physicians (Berardo et al, 1994; Cooper, 1997; Deady et al, 1991; Gums et al, 1999; Klopfer and Einarson, 1990). In any case, the assertive pharmacist is aware at all times that his professional duties are to the patient and is assertive (and persistent) in seeing that the interests of patients are served.

Assertiveness and Employees

Consider the following situation. The manager of a hospital outpatient pharmacy has observed lately that one of the pharmacists has been creating problems. The manager's major concern is that the pharmacist is sometimes rude and abrupt with patients. Today, the manager overhears the pharmacist respond with obvious annoyance to a patient who expressed confusion about how to take her medication. The manager decides to talk privately with the pharmacist about his behavior.

> **MANAGER:** I overheard your conversation with Mrs. Raymond this afternoon when you became impatient with her for not understanding instructions. I was upset because I didn't think you treated her with respect. I want you to treat patients with courtesy and not get so impatient and judgmental with them.

> **PHARMACIST:** Well, she had been complaining about how slow we were and then wouldn't pay attention when I was explaining the directions. I just got fed up.

> **MANAGER:** I know that patients can be irritating, but I want you to treat them with respect.

> **PHARMACIST:** Well, we were so busy then that I just didn't have time to fool around.

> **MANAGER:** I know it gets hectic and you were feeling rushed today, but even then I want you to be more courteous.

> **PHARMACIST:** Well, it would certainly be easier to take time to be nice if you'd get enough pharmacists in here to cover the workload. Furthermore, if you'd train the techs better, they could be a lot more help to us.

> **MANAGER:** Those things may be true, but right now I want to resolve the problem in the way you communicate with patients when you are irritated or hurried. I want you to agree to treat patients with respect, regardless of how busy we get. Will you do that?

> **PHARMACIST:** That's easier said than done.

> **MANAGER:** Will you do it?

Pharmacy managers are responsible not only for how they communicate with patients, but also how other pharmacists and supportive personnel treat patients. They must make clear to all employees what is expected in the way of patient care. In the previous scene, the pharmacy manager used a number of assertive techniques in his conversation with the pharmacist. For one thing, he was specific about how he expected the pharmacist to behave and calmly repeated these expectations (called a "broken-record" response) in spite of the pharmacist's excuses. He would not let himself be dragged off the point. He did not become defensive when the pharmacist attacked his performance as a manager. He might also have said, "I would like to discuss any ideas you might have about improving the training of techs another time, but right now I want to talk about the way you counsel patients." This would have let the pharmacist know that he was willing to listen to specific, constructive suggestions but not before the current problem was resolved.

The pharmacy manager also used appropriate feedback techniques. He told the pharmacist what he had observed about a specific behavior and what he wanted changed without attacking the pharmacist as a person. The manager did not label the pharmacist as being rude or thoughtless. Focusing feedback on what a person does is much less destructive than making personal judgments about him as a person. Such feedback also lets him know exactly what must be changed to improve his performance. The manager discussed the situation privately and soon after the incident occurred. Dealing with such a problem immediately is much more effective than waiting until the annual job performance evaluations or until the problem has become so serious that more drastic action is required.

Many of the same guidelines that are useful in giving negative feedback apply as well to praise. A personal statement, such as telling a clerk, "I really appreciate your willingness to stay late tonight to help out" is more meaningful than a general statement (e.g., "You're a good clerk"). In addition, if positive feedback is an ongoing part of the relationship rather than something that gets written only on job performance evaluation forms, it is more effective. Too often, employees feel that the only time they get any feedback from their bosses is when they have done something wrong, which makes it much harder to accept the negative comments. Finally, your willingness to accept even negative feedback from employees (if it is constructive) can create an atmosphere of mutual respect. In the example above, the pharmacy manager conveyed both an assertive and empathic message when he said, "I know it gets hectic and you were feeling rushed today, but even then I want you to be more courteous." He let the pharmacist know that he understood the feelings of frustration and at the same time insisted that certain standards be met in patient care.

Assertiveness and Employers

It is necessary to be assertive not only with your employees, but with your supervisors as well. We often "do as we are told" rather than identify our goals in communication with supervisors and exercise persistence in pursuing those goals. As health professionals, we sometimes work in situations in which supervisors share neither our professional identities nor our ethical standards for patient care. It is necessary for us, then, to define what the professional standards for pharmacists are and to be assertive in insisting that we must meet those standards, whatever our practice environment.

In addition, we may be faced with a situation in which we receive a negative evaluation or criticism of our performance by a supervisor. None of us enjoys hearing that someone is angry or disappointed with us for what we have done. Yet the criticisms we receive (and what we do in response to them) can lead to improved relationships with others, if we can avoid some common pitfalls in our responses to criticism.

For some of us, our first response to criticism is to counterattack. The attitude is, "So what if I did make a mistake—I've seen you blow it a few times yourself." It is as if we can somehow "even the score" by criticizing the accuser. However, such responses mean we never have to deal with the possibly valid concerns others have about our behavior— we can always change the subject to their problems. In contrast to these aggressive responses, for more passive individuals, the initial response to criticism is to apologize excessively, give excuses, and generally act as if it is a catastrophe if someone is upset with them. Neither a passive nor aggressive response fosters problem solving.

When you are criticized, it is important to distinguish between (a) the truths people tell you about your behavior and (b) the judgments (the "wrong" or "bad" indictments) that they attach to your behavior. Often these judgments are arbitrary and are based on values you do not share. Even when you do agree with your criticizer and think you were wrong, you must separate the foolish or careless thing you did from yourself as a person. The following are five responses that are helpful in various types of situations in which criticism is levied.

Getting Useful Feedback

If the criticism is vague, it is necessary first to find out exactly what happened that led to the criticism. Uncovering the problem provides you with feedback that may be useful to you in improving your performance. Therefore, before reacting to any problem, be certain that you understand the exact nature of the problem. If a patient says that people in your pharmacy don't care about customers, find out exactly what happened that was upsetting and led to this conclusion. To know how to improve your service, you must have specific feedback that points out what changes might be indicated.

Agreeing with Criticism

If you consider the criticism you receive to be valid, the most straightforward response is to acknowledge the mistake. If it is possible to counteract any of the damage, then that is done. In any case, avoid "yes, but..." responses that try to excuse behavior but lead to increased annoyance on the part of the other person. "Yes, I am late for work a lot, but the traffic is so bad" usually leads to an escalation of the conflict ("You'll just have to leave home earlier!"). If you made a mistake or are wrong, acknowledge this without excuses. It also helps to report on efforts being made to implement change so the problem is not repeated.

Disagreeing with Criticism

Often criticism is not justified or is not appropriate because it is too broad, it is a personal attack rather than a criticism of specific behavior; or, it is based on value judgments that you do not agree with. If you consider criticism unfair or unreasonable, it is important to state your disagreement and tell why. For example, you came in late for work this morning and your boss is fuming. During his attack, he says, "You're always late. Nobody around here cares about the patients waiting to get prescriptions filled."

It is important to say to him: "You're right, I was late this morning, and for that I apologize. But it is not true that I am always late. I know I was late a day last month but that is the only other time I can recall being late in the two years I have worked here. And it is not true that I do not care about our patients. I think the way I practice shows them my concern."

Not speaking against something you consider to be a personal injustice or untruth leads to feelings of resentment and a loss of self-esteem for having kept quiet.

Fogging

Fogging involves acknowledging the truth or possible truths in what people tell you about yourself while ignoring completely any judgments they might have implied by what they said. Manuel Smith (1975) outlined this as a basic assertive response to criticism. Let us see how this might apply in a pharmacy situation.

> **SUPERVISOR:** You spent a lot of time talking with that patient about a simple OTC choice.
>
> **PHARMACIST:** You're right. I did.
>
> **SUPERVISOR:** The other pharmacists let clerks do a lot of that sort of stuff.
>
> **PHARMACIST:** You're probably right. They may not spend as much time as I do on OTC consultations.

Such a response allows you to look at possible truths without accepting implied criticisms. The response makes it clear that your own standards guide your behavior without provoking a confrontation with the person levying the criticism.

Delaying a Response

If the criticism takes you by surprise and you are confused about how to respond, give yourself time to think about the problem before responding. Few conflict situations call for an immediate response. If you are too surprised or upset to think clearly about what you want to say, then delay a response. Tell the person: "I want time to think about what you've told me, and then I'd like to sit down with you and try to clear up this problem. Could we discuss the situation this afternoon at the end of my shift?"

Assertiveness and Colleagues

The techniques for assertiveness with employers can also help you be more assertive with your colleagues. For example, the president of your local pharmacy association calls and asks you to serve as chairman of a new committee. You are interested in the committee but are not sure you have the time. Which of the following responses would you choose:

 a. "Well, I'd really like to. I don't know. I guess I could if it doesn't take too much time."
 b. "Why don't you ask Jim? He'd be good. If you can't find anyone else, maybe I could do it."
 c. "I've given enough time to this organization. Everyone always comes to me. Let someone else do some work for a change."
 d. "I'm interested in the committee, but I'm not sure I have time. Let me think about it tonight and I'll call you in the morning with my decision."

Response (d) seems most honest and assertive. We often feel that we must respond immediately to situations. Often the best response is to delay a response. It gives you time to decide what it is you really want to do. When you are facing a decision or when you are embroiled in a conflict, it is often best to say, "I want time to think. I'll get back to you." It is, of course, essential that you do get back to that person and resolve the issue. Response (a) is a wishy-washy "yes." The problem with such a response is that you may say "yes" but never take responsibility for your decision. You may instead blame others for asking too much of you. The yes response, in this situation, was given because you found it difficult to say "no." Response (b) suggests that, if no one else will do it, you will feel that you must do it. You feel responsible for solving the president's problem by identifying someone to chair the committee. If he cannot find someone else, you will then feel obligated. The aggressive response, (c) is often the point a person comes to after a history of passive responses to similar requests. It sounds as if this person has said "yes" frequently in the past, felt overcommitted, and began to blame others for asking rather than taking personal responsibility for having said yes.

Others will make requests of you. It is up to you to say yes or no or to set limits on the extent of your involvement. Let's now imagine a situation in which the president tries to coax or manipulate you into changing a "no" to a "yes" response to his request to chair the committee.

> **PRESIDENT:** You would be perfect for the job. It is extremely important and I must have someone who knows the issues and stays on top of things.

> **PHARMACIST:** I appreciate that, but I won't be able to chair the committee this year.

> **PRESIDENT:** I'll help with the workload. It shouldn't take more than an hour or so a week.

> **PHARMACIST:** That may be true, but I'm not willing to chair the committee right now.

> **PRESIDENT:** Why not? Perhaps there is something we can do to resolve the problems you seem to think will come up in chairing the committee.

> **PHARMACIST:** The decision is really a personal one. I won't be able to chair the committee at this time.

In this instance, the pharmacist again used a "broken record" response. He calmly repeated his "no" response without elaboration and with no rancor at the president's efforts to coax him into changing his mind. If the pharmacist had chosen to do so, he might have given an explanation for his decision, but he is not "obliged" to do so. The danger for passive people in giving an explanation is that they seem to believe that the president must agree that the decision is "justified" before they feel they have the right to say no.

SUMMARY

Assertiveness is a style of response that focuses on resolving conflicts in relationships in an atmosphere of mutual respect. To be assertive, each person must be able to directly and honestly convey: "This is what I think." "This is how I feel about the situation." "This is what I want to have happen." "This is what I am willing to do." This type of communication allows people to stand up for their rights or what they believe in without infringing on the rights of others. You attempt to understand the other person's point of view even when there is disagreement. The focus is on problem solving rather than on turning the conflict into a win–lose situation that damages the relationship.

As a pharmacist, you are faced with numerous changes in your role within the health care system. If you are to lead these changes, to have a hand in shaping your own future, you must be assertive in your communication with the persons you relate to as a pharmacist.

REVIEW QUESTIONS

1. Compare assertiveness with passivity and aggressiveness.
2. In what way(s) should pharmacists be assertive with patients? With physicians? With colleagues?
3. Describe a way in which to handle criticism without losing self-esteem or mutual respect.
4. How can assertiveness be used to resolve conflict?
5. What is "fogging?"

References

Berardo DH, Kimberlin CL, McKenzie LC, Pendergast JF. Community pharmacists' documentation of intervention on drug-related problems of elderly patients. *Journal of Social and Administrative Pharmacy* 11:182–193, 1994.

Cooper J. Consultant pharmacist assessment and reduction of fall risk in nursing facilities. *Consultant Pharmacist* 12: 1294–1298, 1303–1304, 1997.

Deady JE, Lepinski PW, Abramowitz PW. Measuring the ability of clinical pharmacists to effect drug therapy changes in a family practice clinic using prognostic indicators. *Hospital Pharmacy* 26: 93–97, 1991.

Gums JG, Yancey RW, Hamilton CA, Kubilis PS. Randomized, prospective study measuring outcomes after antibiotic therapy intervention by a multidisciplinary consult team. *Pharmacotherapy* 19: 1369–1377, 1999.

Kaplan SH, Greenfield S, Ware JE, Jr. Assessing the effects of physician–patient interactions on the outcomes of chronic disease. *Medical Care* 27: 5110–5127, 1989.

Kimberlin C, Assa M, Rubin D, Zaenger P. Questions elderly patients have about on-going therapy: A pilot study to assist in communication with physicians. *Pharmacy World and Science* 23: 237–241, 2001.

Klopfer JD, Einarson TR. Acceptance of pharmacists' suggestions by prescribers: literature review. *Hospital Pharmacy* 25: 830–832, 834–836, 1990.

Roter D. Patient participation in patient-provider interactions: the effects of patient question-asking on the quality of interactions, satisfaction and compliance. *Health Education Monographs* 5: 281–315, 1977.

Roter DL. Patient question asking in physician-patient interaction. *Health Psychology* 3: 395–409, 1984.

Smith M. *When I Say No, I Feel Guilty.* New York: Dial Press, 1975.

Chapter 8

Interviewing and Assessment

▓ OVERVIEW

Patient assessment is an important aspect of patient care. Determining what patients understand about their medications, how they are taking their medications, how well their medications are working, and problems they perceive with their therapy are key elements to ensuring positive health outcomes. Gaining insight into patient understanding and actions assists pharmacists in planning an appropriate strategy for increasing understanding and appropriate use of medications.

Interviewing is one of the most common methods used in patient assessment. Although interviewing is common in pharmacy practice, the quality of the patient interview is an area that receives little attention by pharmacists. This chapter focuses on ways of improving patient assessment and the interviewing process. It addresses aspects of both informal questioning and the more formal, structured interview. Communication skills discussed include questioning, listening, using silence appropriately, and developing rapport.

Introduction

Pharmacists often must obtain information from patients as part of the patient assessment process. Inquiries range from rather simple requests, such as asking whether a patient is allergic to penicillin, to rather complex problems, such as determining whether a patient is taking a medication properly. Interviewing is an important component in the disease management process because pharmacists obtain information for therapeutic decision making. Effective interviewing also allows pharmacists to evaluate patient adherence to medication regimens by asking appropriate questions. At first glance, this process appears to be rather simple; it is something pharmacists do many times each day. However, research and experience have shown that interviewing is a complex process in need of more attention, because the quality of the information received is not always optimal.

The accuracy, depth, and breadth of information provided by a patient in an interview are influenced by many factors, such as the patient's perception of the interview and the physical environment in which the interview takes place—factors that have been discussed earlier. However, the accuracy of the patient assessment is also influenced by the interviewing process and by the way questions are asked by pharmacists.

One of the first steps in the patient assessment process should be to determine not only what medications patients may take but also what patients already know about their medications and their health-related problems. Determining how much patients know is necessary because patient education strategies vary according on the depth of understanding patients already possess. Patients who are very familiar with their medications have different needs from those who know relatively little. You become more efficient when you can identify those people who need extra counseling. It is inefficient to repeat information that patients already understand. By using an initial assessment technique, you essentially use the patient as a database to determine what information is already mastered. You then fill in the void with the information you think is important for a particular patient.

The process of interviewing goes beyond asking a series of preplanned questions in a certain order. Although this approach may be effective in some aspects of pharmacy care, such as screening for hypertension, it may not be the most appropriate approach in other situations, such as when patients are reluctant to talk about their problems (Bernstein and Bernstein, 1980). The basic skills discussed in this unit can be used in a variety of settings or situations and, if used properly, can greatly enhance the efficiency of the interview and the quality of information obtained.

Components of an Effective Interview

Conducting an effective interview is not a simple process. The interviewing process contains several critical components that should be mastered. The process is somewhat analogous to learning to drive a car. At first, you must learn specific skills, such as using a clutch or gear shift, applying brakes properly, and using the rearview mirror. Once these skills have been learned, the process becomes automatic and rather simple—until you have an accident. Then you must analyze what went wrong with your skills (e.g., you didn't use the turn signal, or you miscalculated your speed on a curve); the driving skill is then corrected or relearned, and you continue on safely. The same is true with effective interviewing. Certain communication and interviewing skills need to be mastered and used or you are likely to have an incomplete or otherwise unproductive interview. The problems in the interviewing process can be minor (e.g., you miss one piece of information) or major (e.g., the patient stomps out of the pharmacy vowing never to return). By considering the elements of effective interviewing in this chapter, you will be able to avoid problems and analyze what went wrong if a problem does arise.

Listening

In general, people are better senders of information than receivers. We have been taught how to improve our verbal and written communication skills, but not our listening skills. Thus, we must concentrate much harder on the listening component of the communication process. Nothing ends an interview faster than having patients realize that you are not listening to them. Although listening skills have been discussed in Chapter 6, listening techniques to use during the interview process are offered in Box 8.1.

Probing

Another important communication skill is learning to ask questions in a way that elicits the most accurate information. This technique is called *probing*. Probing is the use of questions to elicit needed information from patients or to help clarify their problems or concerns. Asking questions seems to be a straightforward task, and it is in most situations. However, several things should be considered before asking a question.

The *phrasing* of the question is important. Patients are often put on the defensive by questions. For instance, "why" type questions can make people feel that they have to justify why they did a certain thing.

Box 8.1 LISTENING TECHNIQUES FOR THE INTERVIEW PROCESS

1. Stop talking. You can't listen while you are talking.
2. Get rid of distractions. These break your concentration.
3. Use good eye contact. That is, look at the other person to help you concentrate and show the other person that you are indeed listening.
4. React to ideas, not to the person. Focus on what is being said and not on whether you like the person.
5. Read nonverbal messages. These may communicate the same or a different message than the one given verbally.
6. Listen to how something is said. The tone of voice and rate of speech also transmit part of the message.
7. Provide feedback to clarify any messages. This also shows that you are listening and trying to understand.

It is usually better to use "what" or "how" type of questions. For example, many people might be defensive if asked "why do you miss doses of medication?" rather than " what causes you to miss doses of medication?"

In addition, the *timing* of the question is important. Several questions in succession may leave the patient with a sense of being interrogated and therefore may raise the level of defensiveness. The patient should be allowed to finish answering the current question before proceeding to the next one. In addition, leading questions should be avoided. These questions strongly imply an expected answer (e.g., "You don't usually forget to take the medication, do you?" or "You take this three times a day with meals, right?"). These questions lead patients to say what they think you want to hear rather than what the truth may be.

To conduct an effective interview, it is important to understand the differences between closed-ended and open-ended questions. A closed-ended question can be answered with either a "yes" or "no" response or with a few words at most. On the other hand, an open-ended question neither limits the patient's response nor induces defensiveness. For example, a closed-ended question would be "Has your doctor told you how to take this medication?" The patient may only respond with a yes and not provide any useful information to you. On the other hand, an example of an open-ended question would be "How has your doctor told you to take this medication?" The phrasing of this question allows patients to state exactly how they perceive that the medication should be taken.

Proper open-ended questions are harder to formulate than closed-ended questions, but they are more crucial in obtaining complete information and in decreasing the patient's defensiveness by conveying a willingness on your part to listen. With an open-ended question you are allowing patients to present information in their own words.

Closed-ended questions reduce the patient's degree of openness and cause the patient to become more passive during the interviewing process because you are doing most of the talking. Closed-ended questions also enable patients to avoid specific subjects and emotional expression. Closed-ended questions can connote an air of interrogation and impersonality. For this reason, closed-ended questions are referred to as "pharmacist-centered questions." Open-ended questions do not require the other person to respond in your frame of reference. Open-ended questions permit open expression and for this reason are sometimes referred to as "patient-centered questions." Closed-ended questions are necessary and are indeed useful; however, open-ended questions are less likely to result in misunderstanding and tend to promote rapport.

You may find a combination of open-ended and closed-ended questions most efficient for you in your practice. Patient encounters may be initiated with an open-ended question, followed by more directed, closed-ended questions. For example, if you want to know whether Mr. Raymond is experiencing bothersome side effects from his antihypertensive medication, you may say, "How have you been feeling since starting this medicine?" or "What things have you noticed since beginning this medication?" If symptoms that may indicate a side effect of the medication are mentioned, follow-up questions are indicated to assess the severity of the adverse effects, such as "How bothersome are these side effects?" If necessary, open-ended questioning can be followed by more direct questions that focus on specific side effects often associated with a particular medication, such as "Do you have trouble sleeping?" "Do you feel weak?" "Do you feel tired?" and so on.

Experience has found that open-ended questions are more effective in assessing patient understanding. The Indian Health Service has developed an effective patient education program that uses a series of open-ended questions during the patient assessment process (Gardner et al, 1991). For new prescriptions, the questions, "What did your doctor tell you the medication is for," "How did your doctor tell you to take the medication," and "What did your doctor tell you to expect," are suggested as a way to structure the assessment of patient understanding of new prescriptions (Gardner et al, 1991). Open-ended questions provide an opportunity for you to assess whether or not the patient understands the key elements of drug therapy (Box 8.2).

> **Box 8.2** KEY ELEMENTS OF DRUG THERAPY
>
> - Purpose of the medication
> - How the medication works
> - Dose/interval
> - Duration of therapy
> - Goals of therapy
> - How effectiveness will be monitored
> - Adverse effects and strategies to deal with these events
> - Drug specific issues

Based on these assessments of patient knowledge, you will be able to develop a strategy to deal with patients' lack of knowledge or their misconceptions about drug use. You may provide additional information, calm their fears, and provide necessary encouragement. You may also give them take-home material and follow up with a phone call in the future.

Whatever the purpose of the patient interview, be aware of when and how you ask a question. The ultimate test is this: Will the question I am about to ask be helpful in understanding the other person's drug therapy needs and problems? Open-ended questions elicit more complete and unabridged information that does not squeeze the patient into your perspective. Open-ended questions convey a willingness to listen. Conversely, closed-ended questions reduce openness, can encourage passivity, and can lead to patient avoidance of emotional expression. Open-ended questions are almost always better than closed-ended questions because they yield more information. Of course, in some situations a simple "yes" or "no" answer will be necessary.

Closed-ended questions help collect specific clinical data efficiently. It takes practice to develop a good questioning technique that uses a combination of both closed- and open-ended questions to move the interview to its conclusion. You need to develop tact when using open-ended questions to prevent patients from wandering off into subject areas that might not be relevant to the situation.

Asking Sensitive Questions

Some questions that you ask patients may be particularly sensitive. Questions assessing adherence, alcohol use, or use of recreational drugs may be difficult to ask. Assessment of effects (including side effects) of medications that relate to sexual functioning or sexually transmitted diseases may also require a diplomatic approach. There are a number of techniques that can make such questions easier to ask.

Before asking a question on a sensitive topic, let the patient know that the behaviors or problems you are asking about are common. If you acknowledge that "everyone" has similar problems, it makes the issue seem less threatening. For example, saying to a patient, "It is very difficult to take a medication consistently, day after day. Nearly everyone will miss a dose of medication once in a while," before asking specific questions about adherence can make it seem safe for patients to admit to difficulty adhering to a medication regimen. Patients do not fear that you will judge them harshly for missing doses of medication if you preface your question with an accepting statement. Gardner and colleagues (1995) refer to these remarks as "universal statements." Examples of universal statements that they identify include, "This is a very common concern. . .," "Frequently my patients have difficulty. . . ," and "Everybody has trouble with...."

Another technique for reducing the threat of sensitive questions is to ask whether the situation has ever occurred and then ask about the current situation. For example, if you decide that you must assess use of recreational drugs, you may phrase the question in the following way: "Other types of drugs, such as marijuana, are commonly used. People might use marijuana to relax or with friends at a party. Have you at any time in your life smoked marijuana?" If the answer is yes, the follow-up question might be "To put things in a more recent time frame, have you smoked marijuana during the past year?" Questions about frequency of use and use of other drugs could follow. A similar process could be used to obtain precise information on adherence to a regimen, such as use of antiretroviral agents in which strict adherence is important. Asking first whether the patient has ever missed a dose of a medication and then progressing to estimates of the number of doses missed in the last week may make the information the patient provides more reliable.

In addressing sensitive issues, use of simple, clear-cut questions and a matter-of-fact manner is critical. The way you phrase the question and your tone of voice should be no different for a question on alcohol consumption than for a question on the use of an OTC product.

In structuring the interview, it helps to embed more threatening topics among less threatening topics and to ask more "personal" questions later in the interview. For example, questions about alcohol consumption may be better accepted by the patient when such questions follow questions about caffeine consumption.

When patients seem reluctant to address an issue, it helps to discuss the reason why you are asking a particular question. A statement such as "People often do not think of alcohol as a drug, but there are many medications that can interact with alcohol. I ask about alcohol use so that I can help you prevent problems with the medications you take." If patients understand the reason for a question, they are more likely to respond honestly. If they do not know the reason, they may make assumptions about why questions are being asked. Unfortunately, the assumptions they make may be more damaging than the truth. In any case, before asking **any** question, and especially one that may be sensitive, be sure that the question is necessary and that you have a clear need for the information in your efforts to help the patient.

Use of Silence

Another skill that you need to learn to be an effective interviewer is the art of using silence appropriately. During an interview, there are times when neither you nor the patient will speak, especially in the early moments. You must learn to treat these pauses as a necessary part of the process and not be uncomfortable with them. Many times, the patient needs time to think about or react to the information you have provided or the question you have asked. Interrupting the silence destroys the opportunity for the patient to think about this material. On the other hand, the pause might be due to the fact that the patient did not understand the question completely. In this situation, the question should be restated or rephrased. At the same time, too much silence when a patient is expressing feelings, such as fear or depression, may be interpreted by the patient as rejection. In this case, the patient may be seeking an indication that you understand the concerns expressed.

In any event, avoid the temptation to fill empty spaces in the interview with unnecessary talk. In fact, some studies have found that the more the "talk ratio" is in favor of the person being interviewed (i.e., the patient does more of the talking), the more likely that the interview will be successful. Thus, the patient should be able to relax and be allowed time to think during the necessary pauses in the interview process.

Establishing Rapport

Successful interviews are marked by a high degree of rapport between the two parties. Rapport is built mainly on mutual consideration and respect. You can aid this process by using good eye contact, by using a sincere, friendly greeting, by being courteous during the discussion, and by not stereotyping or prejudging the patient. Each patient must be seen as a unique individual. Patient perception of you, the pharmacist, will influence their relationship with you. Thus, it is critical that you initiate the interaction in a friendly, professional manner.

Interviewing as a Process

Proper planning and sequencing of the interview are essential in carrying out an effective patient assessment. Before an interview is started,

Box 8.3 SUMMARY OF INTERVIEW CONSIDERATIONS

- Type of information
- Type of environment
- Starting the interview
- Ending the interview

several decisions must be made regarding how it will be structured (Box 8.3). The type of approach usually depends on the type of information desired and the environment available for it.

Type of Information

Before the interview begins, determine the amount and type of information desired. In other words, what exactly do you want to accomplish? For example, if you need to find out specific pieces of information, you will want to have more control over the interview process. This is referred to as the *directed-interview approach*. However, if the outcome is unknown or somewhat ambiguous, you need to use a more *nondirected approach*. This approach allows the interview to become more free flowing; the points of discussion are raised by the patient rather than by you. When you use a nondirected approach, you hope the problem or concern will surface, allowing you to deal with it. In the nondirected approach, open-ended questions should be used more frequently than closed-ended questions. However, even in the directed approach you can ask an initial open-ended question to assess patient understanding, as discussed earlier.

Type of Environment

Planning for the interview must include consideration of the type of environment available. The environment is critical, because one of the fundamental principles of interviewing is to provide as much privacy as possible. Research has shown that the degree of privacy is related to many critical outcomes of the interview process (e.g., the level of patient understanding of the information provided and the degree of adherence with the treatment regimen). As the privacy of the setting improves, the amount of information retained by the patient increases, along with the likelihood that the patient will take the prescribed medication appropriately (Beardsley et al, 1977). Privacy also allows both you and the patient to express personal concerns, to ask difficult questions, to listen more effectively, and to share honest opinions. Unfortunately, the setting of the interview in many pharmacies—over a busy prescription counter or in other areas where distractions abound—is not always optimal.

Before beginning the interview, try to reduce interruptions as much as possible. A partition at the end of the prescription counter, a special room, or a consulting area can provide the necessary privacy.

Starting the Interview

After considering the type of environment available and the type of information desired, start the interview by greeting patient by name and by introducing yourself if you do not know him or her. This helps establish rapport. You should also state the purpose of the interview, outline what will happen during the interview, and put the patient at ease. The purpose of the interview should be stated in terms of the benefit to the patient. The amount of time needed, the subjects to be covered, and the final outcome should be mentioned so that the patient has a clear understanding of the process. For example, a pharmacist seeing a patient for the first time might say:

"Hello, Mr. Pearson, I'm Jane Bradley, the pharmacist [the introduction]. Since you are new to our pharmacy, I would like to ask you a few quick questions about the medications you are now taking [the subjects to be covered]. This will take about 5 to 10 minutes [the amount of time needed] and will allow me to create a drug profile so that I can keep track of all the medications that you are taking. This will help us identify potential problems with new medications that might be prescribed for you [the purpose/outcome]."

Such a beginning allows you to define the limits and expectations of the interview. After the interview is started, the following suggestions will help you to conduct a more efficient interview:

1. Avoid making recommendations during the information-gathering phases of the interview. Such recommendations prevent the patient from giving you all the needed information and can interfere with your ability to grasp the "big picture" of patient need.

2. Similarly, do not jump to conclusions or rapid solutions without hearing all the facts.

3. Do not shift from one subject to another until each subject has been followed through.

4. Guide the interview using a combination of open-ended and closed-ended questions.

5. Similarly, keep your goals clearly in mind, but do not let them dominate how you go about the interview.

6. Determine the patient's ability to learn specific information in order to guide you in your presentation of the material. Reading ability, language proficiency, and vision or hearing impairment all would influence the techniques you use in interviewing and counseling a patient.

7. Maintain objectivity by not allowing the patient's attitudes, beliefs, or prejudices to influence your thinking.

8. Use good communication skills, especially the probing, listening, and feedback components.

9. Be aware of the patient's nonverbal messages, because these signal how the interview is progressing.

10. Depending on your relationship with the patient, move from general to more specific questions and from less personal to more personal subjects. This may remove some of the patient's initial defensiveness.

11. Note taking should be as brief as possible.

Ending the Interview

Bringing the interview to a close is often more difficult than starting the interview. It is a crucial part of the interview process because a person's evaluation of the entire interview and your performance may be based on the final statements. People seem to remember best what was said last. Therefore, care should be taken not to end the interview abruptly or to rush the patient out the door.

If you have provided important information to the patient, you should determine whether or not the patient understood the material correctly at the end of the interaction. Telling a patient "I want to make sure I have explained everything clearly. Summarize for me the most important things to remember about this new medicine?" will allow patients to reflect what they heard and understood. Other simple open-ended questions are "When you get home, how are you going to take this medication?" or "What side effects are you going to look for when taking this medication?"

To conclude the interview, briefly summarize the key information provided by the patient. A summary allows both parties the opportunity to review exactly what has been discussed and helps to clarify any misunderstanding. It is essential that both people agree about what has been said. A summary sets the stage for future patient contact and expectations that you both have of one another. A summary also tactfully hints to the patient that the interview is ending. In conjunction with a summary, you can use nonverbal cues to indicate to the patient that the interview is over. For instance, you could get up from the chair or change your stance in such a way that indicates that you need to move on. A simple closed-ended question may be helpful, such as "Do you have any further questions?" or a statement such as "I've enjoyed talking with you. If you think of something you forgot to mention or have questions when you get home, please give me a call" may also be useful. The ending of the interview is a good time for you to reassure the patient about a particular problem. However, this should not be false assurance, such as "Everything is going to turn out okay" or "Don't worry about it." Rather, you should state, "I will try to help things get better for you" along with specific action or follow-up you will implement. Tell the patient when you will contact him or her and how (e.g., by telephone) in order to make sure that a problem identified has been resolved and that the patient is responding well to any therapeutic changes that have been made.

With a new prescription, follow-up is also important to identify and resolve possible problems early in treatment. Waiting until a refill visit to find out how a patient is doing with a new prescription is often not the most timely or effective way to monitor response to a medication. Before terminating the patient interview, you should reflect on whether the goals of the interview were accomplished and what should be done if they were not. After the patient has left, assess in your own mind what went well and what could have been done differently to help you continue to improve your interviewing skills. Finally, key information must be documented as part of the patient record. The information that should be documented from a patient interview is described later in this chapter.

Interviewing in Pharmacy Practice

Interviews in pharmacy practice are often thought of in terms of complete medication history interviews. However, if an interview is thought of as a process of obtaining information from patients to assess potential medication-related problems, then there are a number of activities that pharmacists engage in that can be thought of as interviewing. Assessing the health problems a patient presents before making an OTC recommendation is a targeted interview. Evaluating a patient's response to treatment and perceived problems related to medication therapy during a refill visit is another example of an interview. The specific questions that are asked may vary somewhat because the purpose of the interview varies, but the skills involved in gathering information from patients to make an assessment of patient problems and needs remain the same.

In assessing medication therapy, such as in a medication history interview, it is necessary to ensure that you have a complete list of medications being taken, including prescriptions, OTCs, herbal products, and other complementary and alternative medicines. For each medication, an assessment is made of (a) the patient's perception of the purpose of the medication, (b) the way the medication is actually being used by the patient, (c) patient's perceived effectiveness (along with specific information on indicators of effectiveness derived from physician reports to the patient or patient self-monitoring of response) of the medication, and (d) problems the patient perceives with therapy.

It is also important to ask patients about health problems that they have been experiencing or that they have been diagnosed with for which they are not currently being treated with medication. You want to uncover health problems that should be brought to the attention of providers but, for whatever reasons, have not been discussed. Perhaps the patient does not consider the problem "important" enough or perhaps the costs associated with office visits and treatments are of concern. Fears related to an imagined diagnosis may prevent patients from seeking care. In other cases, a patient may have received a diagnosis (e.g., type 2 diabetes) that is being treated by means other than medication (e.g., diet and exercise). In addition, patients may have received a diagnosis and have been prescribed a medication for a chronic condition that they decided on their own either not to use or to discontinue. Medication-related problems include not only problems with medications being taken, but also drug therapy that is needed but is not being received by the patient.

Let's examine an example of an interview in a community pharmacy setting. A new patient, Robert Evans, comes to the pharmacy and presents a prescription for hydrochlorothiazide. Pharmacist Ed Robinson initiates a brief interview with the patient.

ED: Hello. Are you Robert Evans?

MR. EVANS: Yes

ED: Mr. Evans, I'm Ed Robinson, the pharmacist here. I would like to sit down with you and talk about the medications you currently take. This can help us identify problems you might be having with your drug therapy. We can talk while the technician is filling your prescription. Do you have about 10 minutes?

MR. EVANS: Sure. I was going to wait for my prescription anyway.

ED: Let's start with the prescription you brought in today. What has your doctor told you about this medicine?

MR. EVANS: Dr. Carter told me I have high blood pressure. This isn't the first prescription for this HCTZ (hydrochlorothiazide) medicine though. I've been taking it about 3 years. My old prescription ran out of refills. Dr. Carter gave me a new one today.

Ed: When were you first diagnosed with high blood pressure?

Mr. Evans: About 3 years ago. I don't remember what my blood pressure was but the doc said it was high.

Ed: Are you taking any other medications for your high blood pressure?

Mr. Evans: No, just the one.

Ed: How well has the HCTZ medication worked for you?

Mr. Evans: It has done the trick. Dr. Carter says I'm doing great.

Ed: That's good to hear. What was your blood pressure today when you saw Dr. Carter?

Mr. Evans: 125/85. I take my blood pressure myself every day, and it always stays around that.

Ed: It's a great idea to keep track of your own blood pressure. How often do you see Dr. Carter to have your blood pressure checked by him?

Mr. Evans: I see him every 6 months. At first it was every couple of months. But he said I am doing so well now, he doesn't have to see me as often.

Ed: Tell me, what problems have you had with this medication?

Mr. Evans: I haven't had any problems.

Ed: Have you noticed any side effects or symptoms you think are related to the medication?

Mr. Evans: I haven't had any side effects. I really haven't had any problems with the medication.

Ed: I'm glad to hear that. How have you been taking the HCTZ? Describe a typical schedule for using the medication.

Mr. Evans: I take it when I eat breakfast. I fill up one of those weekly pill containers every Sunday and keep it beside the cereal in the cupboard.

Ed: It's sometimes difficult to take a medication every day, day after day. How often would you say you miss a dose in a typical week?

Mr. Evans: I never miss. Last time I forgot to take it I had gone to a restaurant for breakfast and I forgot it that morning. But that hardly ever happens.

Ed: Are there other things you do to help you control your high blood pressure?

Mr. Evans: Dr. Carter put me on a diet and exercise program. I've lost over 50 pounds in the past couple of years. I don't eat a lot of salt either.

ED: It sounds as if you're really doing what you need to do to keep your blood pressure down. Do you have any questions or concerns about your medicine or your high blood pressure?

MR. EVANS: No. I think I've been doing fine. I've gotten used to taking a pill every day.

ED: If any concerns do come up in the future, please let me know. Next, let me ask about other prescription medications you might currently be taking?

MR. EVANS: I don't take anything else. One drug is all I take.

ED: I see. Let me switch to over-the-counter products that you can buy without a prescription.

MR. EVANS: I don't take anything. Maybe Tylenol (acetaminophen) once a year for a headache. Doc told me not to take anything for a cold without checking with him or a pharmacist. I don't like taking drugs, so I don't use that stuff you can buy in a grocery store.

ED: Any vitamins or herbal products?

MR. EVANS: Nope.

ED: Do you have any health concerns or other conditions a doctor has told you about that you are not treating with medication?

MR. EVANS: None. I'm healthy except for the high blood pressure.

ED: That's good to hear. Do you have any allergies, especially reactions to medications?

MR. EVANS: No, no allergies at all.

At this point, the pharmacist might conclude the interview by thanking the patient for taking the time to answer questions, by making sure there is not another issue related to drug therapy that the patient might want to discuss, and by making himself available by telephone or in person if the patient wants to discuss drug therapy or any health concerns in the future.

In this example, the goal of the questions the pharmacist asked Mr. Evans was to establish a medication record along with a record of current medical conditions. In addition, the pharmacist sought to obtain the information needed to assess the effectiveness of and problems with the treatment of current conditions. The interview was limited, focusing on information needed to assess problems with current therapy and to uncover health problems that are not being treated with medications. For the medications the patient was currently taking, assessment focused on:

- Patient understanding of purpose
- Actual patterns of use and problems with use

- Perceived effectiveness along with specific information from physician monitoring and patient self-monitoring that could provide additional "evidence" that the pharmacist could use to assess patient response to treatment
- Patient perceptions of problems with therapy

Patient-perceived problems may include side effects experienced, cost concerns, inconvenience of dosing schedules, and so on. Phrasing a very open-ended question on problems allows patients to discuss anything they might perceive as problematic. More direct or closed-ended follow-up questions on specific issues of concern, such as whether the patient has experienced symptoms that may indicate adverse reactions to the medication, may be indicated to ensure that these problems are given particular attention and that information about such issues are not overlooked.

While in the above example the pharmacist made the judgment to conduct a focused, brief interview, more extensive data gathering may be desirable or a series of interviews over time may be conducted to obtain a more complete picture of the patient's medical conditions and treatment needs. For example, a more intensive interviewing process has been described as a key component of the Pharmacist's Work-up of Drug Therapy (Cipolle et al, 1998). This work-up is designed to thoroughly evaluate a patient's drug-related needs and drug therapy problems. Information is obtained in a number of areas, including demographics and family history, past medical history, current medical problems, allergies and adverse drug reactions, lifestyle issues related to health, immunization history, a medication record of current and recent past medication use, and a review of systems for thorough assessment of drug-related needs of the patient.

A benefit of conducting an in-depth interview is that you will be better able to determine a patient's quality of life (QOL), which is a very important measure of therapeutic success. Patients' QOL beliefs may help you determine how they define therapeutic success. To you, the therapy may appear to be working, whereas your patients may think it is not, since it has not improved their ability to engage in the activities they wish to engage in. Using probing questions related to QOL functioning during the interview process allows you to explore these important factors.

Documenting Interview Information

The documentation process is crucial as a way of ensuring continuity of care to patients. The information documented in a note becomes the "institutional memory" of the care that has been provided to patients.

This will assist in your own follow-up care as well as communicate to colleagues about the care you have provided to a particular patient. Such communication is essential to the functioning of a health care team.

A format for documentation that is familiar to health care professionals is the SOAP note. SOAP is an acronym for subjective, objective, assessment, and plan. Subjective information is that information reported by the patient or patient caregiver, such as symptom experience or self-report of adherence. Objective information is that provided by a lab test or physical exam. If a pharmacist, as part of an interview with a hypertensive patient, takes the patient's blood pressure, for example, this might be documented as objective information. The "assessment" section includes a description of any medication-related problem identified during the interview. For example, a problem may be lack of therapeutic response secondary to reported nonadherence. The assessment should be as specific as possible to lead logically to the plan to resolve the problem (the "P" portion of the SOAP note). For example, nonadherence caused by inability to pay for the prescription requires a different intervention plan from nonadherence caused by forgetting doses.

By the same token, if you obtained information that indicated that the patient was responding well to treatment and had no problems with a medication regimen, this information should be noted and the assessment documented that no problems were identified. This serves to document that the assessment was made. Lack of information on a regimen could be interpreted by a third party to mean that the pharmacist asked no questions about that regimen and an assessment was not made. To make sure communication with colleagues is unambiguous, document findings that indicate appropriate use, adequate response, and no problems with the regimen.

Once the assessment of a problem is made, based on the subjective and objective information included in the note, the plan should detail the actions to be taken to resolve the problem. The plan should include both an intervention plan and a monitoring plan. These plans must be specific. Specify action that will be taken by you, the date the action will be taken, and when follow-up with the patient will occur. For example, an intervention may require a consultation with a prescribing physician for a change in therapy. Document when the physician will be contacted, how (e.g., by phone), what will be recommended, and how the change in therapy will be initiated. The description of the initiation of a change should specify the new regimen as well as who will inform and educate the patient on the changes in therapy. In addition, the plan would document when follow-up with the patient will be initiated to assess the effects of any changes or recommendations made to improve therapy.

Interviewing Using the Telephone

Many times you need to collect information from patients by telephone. In light of the importance of the telephone, you should strive to maximize its effective use. Effective telephone skills can also help create a positive image for your pharmacy and lend support to your professional credibility. In addition, proficient telephone communication can contribute to personnel productivity and ultimately to the professional success of your pharmacy. The following should be considered during this type of interaction:

1. Cue yourself to smile before you pick up the telephone. Your friendly attitude will be transmitted through the tone, pitch, volume, and inflection of your voice.
2. If at all possible, answer the telephone or have a fellow employee answer it within the first three or four rings.
3. Identify the pharmacy and yourself, providing both your name and position (e.g., "Professional Pharmacy, Jane Jones speaking. May I help you?"). Although it may appear burdensome to identify yourself fully to every caller, keep in mind that each call may represent the first contact the caller has with you and your pharmacy. Even if it is not the first contact, each call is a uniquely important communication for the caller and should be given your full attention.
4. Give your full attention to the call. Perhaps nothing is more irritating to callers than to be given the impression that they are competing for your attention.
5. Ask for the caller's name and use the name in the conversation, particularly at the conclusion of the call. Not only does this reduce possible confusion and error, but by asking for and using the caller's name, you project a more personal, empathic attitude.
6. If you must place the caller on hold (for a short time only), ask, "May I put you on hold while I look up your prescription?" In these circumstances, it is important that you do the following:
   a. Tell callers why you want to put them on hold.
   b. Ask whether they would mind waiting a brief time or would prefer to call back (if appropriate).
   c. On returning to the telephone, say, "Thank you for waiting."
7. At the conclusion of the call, end it graciously (e.g., "Thank you for calling").
8. Finally, if possible, allow the caller to hang up first. This allows the caller time to remember that extra request. It also projects in a subtle manner your sincere desire to listen.

Besides receiving telephone calls, many times you must call physicians or other health care professionals to obtain additional information regarding a patient. The following suggestions may help make these calls more efficient.

1. Before you pick up the receiver, be sure you have any and all information related to the call readily available. Prescription, patient, and other relevant information should be obtained before your telephone conversation starts.

2. Before you pick up the receiver, determine with whom you need to speak to achieve your goal for calling.

3. Most important, before you pick up the receiver ask yourself, "Is this call necessary?"

4. Identify yourself, your position, and the pharmacy first. Then ask (if it is not already provided to you) for the same information from the person who has answered your call.

5. Immediately after introducing yourself, state in clear, concise terms the reason for your call. Be assertive! Do not begin by apologizing ("sorry to bother you"). You have already decided that the call is necessary.

6. If the nature of your call dictates that it will exceed more than a couple of minutes, ask the person if they have time to talk with you for a few minutes.

7. Conclude the conversation with a sincere "thank you."

SUMMARY

Conducting patient assessment is a complex process that at times is difficult to master because it involves interactions between two persons. No two interactions are exactly the same, because the sequence of events and the people involved are never exactly the same. Interviews require different levels of flexibility based on the needs of the patient; they also require some type of structure to ensure a time-efficient, clear transmission of information between you and the patient. To conduct a successful interview, certain communication skills need to be mastered. If the two parties are not communicating well, the entire interview process can break down, and the possibility of future positive interactions between the patient and pharmacist can be jeopardized. You must learn how to ask open-ended questions, to transmit information clearly, listen effectively, provide feedback, use silence, and develop rapport. Development of these skills takes time. In addition to using good communication skills, you must realize how to structure the interview. The type of environment, the type of approach, and how to start and how to end the interview are critical to the interview process.

The first step in improving the interview process is to realize that the effective use of these skills leads to a more productive interview. Evaluate each interview by asking such questions as "Did the patient appear to be relaxed and open?" or "Did I check to see if the patient understood me correctly?" Such an analysis reveals some interesting things and points to possible areas of improvement.

The interview is a dynamic process that can always be improved. You cannot rest on previous successes, because many things in the process can be improved. At the same time, don't worry about saying the wrong thing or putting your foot in your mouth. Most patients are forgiving, and relationships can be salvaged even after a negative encounter. The key is to identify what went wrong, correct it, and move on to the next interview.

REVIEW QUESTIONS

1. What are the critical components of an effective interview?
2. Why are people better senders of messages than receivers?
3. What are the differences between open-ended and closed-ended questions, and when should each be used?
4. What are five techniques that improve telephone productivity?

References

Beardsley RS, Johnson CA, Wise G. Privacy as a factor in patient counseling. *Journal of the American Pharmaceutical Association* NS17:366, 1977.

Bernstein L, Bernstein RS. *Interviewing: A Guide for Health Professionals*. New York: Appleton-Century-Crofts, 1980.

Cipolle RJ, Strand LM, Morley PC. *Pharmaceutical Care Practice*. New York: McGraw-Hill, 1998.

Gardner MG, Boyce RW, Herrier RN. *Pharmacist–Patient Consultation Program: An Interactive Approach to Verify Patient Understanding*. New York: Pfizer-Roerig, 1991.

Gardner MG, Boyce RW, Herrier RN. *Pharmacist–Patient Consultation Program, Unit 3: Counseling to Enhance Compliance*. New York: Pfizer-Roerig, 1995.

Part III
Putting It All Together

The final section of this textbook focuses on how to apply the skills described in Parts I and II to actual patient and practice situations. The first chapter in this section (Chapter 9) describes the most common reasons why patients, in general, do not take their medications correctly and how pharmacists can enhance patient outcomes using effective communication skills. Chapters 10 and 11 discuss how to apply these skills to specific patient populations, since different approaches and sensitivities are needed for different types of patients. The key is to be aware of special needs and general characteristics of specific patient populations without stereotyping individuals or making gross assumptions.

Chapter 12 deals with ethical issues to place interpersonal interaction in the context of appropriate and inappropriate behavior. Experience has shown that how and why pharmacists interact with others (as viewed from an ethical framework) influences their effectiveness in working with patients, health care providers, and other pharmacists.

Toward the end of Part III, several examples are provided to illustrate how the various skills and strategies can be used to enhance patient care. Readers are encouraged to develop their own strategies to deal with these examples. As a guide, the following sequence of activities has been shown to be effective in dealing with communication issues: being aware of the various communication elements (what are these elements, which ones are most important, how do we use them, which approach is best), practicing these skills (actually using these skills), and assessing the approach (what went well, what needs to be improved). After this assessment, a new sequence should follow: awareness (what should be done differently next time), practice (conducting the new strategy), and assessment (did it work this time, what could be done differently next time). Many times, this sequence needs to be followed by another cycle of awareness–practice–assessment, and so on, until individuals feel that they have met their goals. It is hoped that the reader appreciates the fact that communication skill development is an ongoing process.

Chapter 9

Ensuring Better Patient Outcomes

▓ OVERVIEW

This chapter presents techniques to help ensure better patient outcomes by building better patient understanding about medication therapy and promoting better patient adherence to treatment regimens. In the delivery of patient care, pharmacists need to develop strategies to assess patient knowledge and to determine possible reasons for lack of adherence with treatment. These techniques use specific skills discussed in previous chapters. The goal of ensuring better patient outcomes must focus on meeting the unique needs of individual patients.

Introduction

A well-known physician once approached his colleagues with this admonition: "Keep watch also on the fault of patients which often makes them lie about taking of things prescribed." Hippocrates said this over 2000 years ago! His comment was based on his experience with patients who lie about how they take their prescribed treatments.

Unfortunately, concern about how patients actually use their prescribed medications continues to this day.

Lack of patient adherence to medication therapy remains a major health issue, according to an Institute of Medicine report (IOM, 2001). The exact rate of adherence to medication regimens is unclear because researchers in this area define and measure adherence differently. For example, some researchers use indirect methods (they interview patients and family members or have patients keep diaries), whereas others use more direct methods (assessing blood or urine levels of medication). Some researchers define adherence as taking medication within 1 hour of prescribed time, whereas others are more lenient by defining adherence as taking the medication within 24 hours of prescribed time. Regardless of definition and measurement, adherence rates are well below 100%. The general consensus is that adherence rates for long-term therapy tend to be about 50%. The exact cost of nonadherence is also unclear because it affects so many aspects of personal life. It often makes a direct impact on patient health, which, in turn, can result in increased emergency room and physician visits, increased hospitalizations, decreased productivity in the work place, and premature death and disability.

Numerous reasons explain why adherence to medication regimens is less than optimal. Some reasons are related to patients; some are related to health care providers; and others evolve from the health care delivery system, such as issues related to insurance, access to medications, and economic concerns. Other reasons for nonadherence include patient perception of medications and the value of following treatment plans as prescribed. Experience and research have shown that patient **perception** of the severity of the illness and the value of treatment and not necessarily the **actual** severity determines the likelihood of adherence. Many patients are afraid to take medications, whereas some rely too heavily on medications and take more than prescribed.

Reasons for nonadherence can be divided into two categories: intentional nonadherence and inadvertent nonadherence. *Inadvertent nonadherence* typically involves forgetting to take medications at prescribed times. *Intentional nonadherence* involves decisions that a patient has made to alter a medication regimen or discontinue drug therapy (permanently or temporarily), such as not taking the medication because of an uncomfortable side effect or skipping doses of a medication that should not be taken with alcohol before going to a party. As discussed in the text that follows, pharmacists would use different approaches to resolve problems related to inappropriate use of medications, depending on the underlying nature of or cause of the nonadherence.

It is beyond the scope of this book to explore the multiple critical issues surrounding patient adherence. The goal of this chapter is to focus on how effective communication skills can enhance patient adherence with medications. In other words, the skills and strategies that pharmacists can use to enhance adherence and ensure better patient outcomes is discussed here. Evidence suggests that enhanced patient–pharmacist interaction improves patient adherence with drug therapy (Hepler and Strand, 1990; Hill, 1989; McKenney, 1990). When pharmacists spend time counseling patients in a meaningful way, patients achieve better outcomes.

Assessing Patient Understanding and Behavior

To enhance patient adherence, first collect information about patient beliefs, understandings, and actual medication use. To do this, use some of the techniques described in Chapter 8, which focus on effective interviewing. It is more efficient to assess patient understanding before conducting counseling interventions. You should determine the level of patient understanding before offering already understood information that wastes time. Counseling time could then be devoted to filling in gaps or correcting misconceptions. Box 9.1 contains open-ended questions that may help assess what a patient understands about his or her antihypertensive regimen.

If a regimen involves more complex behaviors, such as properly using a metered-dose inhaler, the pharmacist must also directly observe the patient administering the medication to effectively assess understanding and appropriate use.

Assessing Understanding of Related Health Issues

To ensure better outcomes, you need to assess patients' other health-related issues. When taking medical histories, determine what other prescription and nonprescription medications patients are taking. In addition, identify their perceptions about their health and medicines, since perceptions affect adherence behavior. You can then correct misperceptions and reinforce correct perceptions. Follow-up questions may include the following:

1. How do you feel about having to take this medication?
2. What do you think will happen to your health if you don't take the medicine as prescribed?

As noted in previous chapters, to be most effective you need to do more than simply tell patients about their medications, you must ask for feedback to make sure they understand your message. Using open-ended questions (how, when, where, what, and why) during patient counseling provides an opportunity for patients to share their under-

---

Box 9.1 QUESTIONS TO ASSESS PATIENT UNDERSTANDING

Assessing Understanding of Medication Purpose

1. What did your doctor tell you about this medicine?
2. What exactly is your medicine supposed to do?
3. What problem has caused you to need this medicine?

Assessing Future Behavior (for New Prescriptions)

1. When do you plan to take your high blood pressure medicine?
2. What would be convenient times for you to take your medicine?
3. How should you be storing this medicine?
4. What exactly does your dosage instructions per day mean to you?
5. How long are you going to be taking this medicine?
6. What did your doctor tell you to do if you missed a dose?
7. What special instructions or precautions were you given?

Assessing Past Behavior (for Ongoing Therapy)

1. How have you been taking the high blood pressure medication?
2. What habits have you had to change since you started taking this medication?
3. Have you missed any doses of your medication this past week? (If yes), How many doses did you miss? What caused you to miss doses?

Assessing Medication Effectiveness

1. How do you know if your blood pressure medication is working?
2. How often does your doctor check your blood pressure?
3. How often do you check your blood pressure yourself?
4. What was your blood pressure reading the last time it was checked?

Assessing Potential Medication Problems

1. What problems have you experienced with this medication?
2. What side effects, if any, have you experienced since you started taking this medicine?
3. What effects are you supposed to watch out for?

---

standing of their particular situation. After listening to patients, you will have a more accurate assessment of their understanding and will be able to fill in gaps of knowledge and reinforce salient points. Using a combination of closed-ended and open-ended questions, you will be able to direct the conversation and at the same time provide an opportunity for patients to articulate their perceptions and concerns.

False Assumptions About Patient Understanding and Medication Adherence

As a pharmacist, you are in a strong position to help patients avoid medication-related problems. To do this, you must have a clear picture of what medications patients take, how they take them, and other information. You should not make general assumptions nor take for granted that patients understand all the aspects of their drug therapy. The following are some common issues that should be kept in mind.

1. Do not assume that physicians have already discussed with patients the medications they prescribe. In fact, one study found that physicians frequently omit critical information (Svarstad, 1986). This study found that instruction for frequency of use was given only 17% of the time during physician office visits. Clear instructions on duration of use were given only 10% of the time.

2. Do not assume that patients understand all information given. Experience has shown that even seemingly straightforward label directions like "take one tablet every 6 hours" is interpreted by a large percentage of patients to mean that they are supposed to take only three doses a day during waking hours. In addition, research has shown that between 35% and 92% of patients do not understand information given to them and about 40% of information learned is soon forgotten (Ley, 1985).

3. Do not assume that if patients understand what is required, they will be able to take the medication correctly. Implementing a new medication regimen requires a change in behavior, which may be difficult. Anyone who has tried to change old habits or implement new ones—a new diet or exercise regimen, for example—knows how hard that can be. Dealing with behavior change requires that you know something about the patient's lifestyle, as well as work, personal, and professional atmosphere, and support and coping mechanisms. Then you can address these in your counseling interventions (Ell, 1986). Some pharmacists believe that if they tell a patient about a medication regimen, it becomes an important priority for that patient. For most people, taking medications becomes an interruption in their busy lives.

4. Do not assume that when patients do not take their medications correctly that they "don't care," "aren't motivated," "lack intelligence," or "can't remember." These assumptions prevent you from focusing on the real problems causing nonadherence. Many patients want to take their medications correctly but are not able to manage this owing to a variety of reasons that are discussed later in this chapter.

5. Do not assume that once patients start taking their medications correctly they will continue to take them correctly in the future. You need to reinforce key messages during your subsequent patient counseling sessions. Experience has shown that once reinforcement stops, patients often stop taking their medications correctly. In addition, some patients become "intelligent non-compliers" where they are sophisticated enough to monitor drug effects and start and stop taking medications as they feel is needed. This phenomenon of intelligent noncompliance is often found among those on chronic medications (Lasagna, 1992). The challenge is to help motivate patients to take their medications correctly when there is no apparent harm for not doing so.

6. Do not assume that physicians routinely monitor patient medication use and will thus intervene if medication problems exist. Because many patients visit multiple physicians, physician office records are often incomplete. In addition, physicians vary greatly in their skills in assessing patient adherence.

7. Do not assume that, if patients are having problems, they will ask direct questions or volunteer information. You cannot be lulled into complacency by thinking that if patients have problems they will contact you. This assumption ignores the fact that patients may be embarrassed to admit they are having problems or may not even realize that they have a problem. You must initiate interaction by asking the open-ended questions discussed earlier.

Techniques to Improve Patient Understanding

After you have assessed patient understanding of their medications, you can enhance patient adherence to treatment regimens by filling in the information gaps with easy-to-understand language. Experience has shown the following strategies to be effective.

1. Examine your own attitude toward patient counseling in specific situations. What is your role in this encounter? Do you have enough time to counsel the patient? What does the patient really need?

2. Emphasize key points. Telling patients beforehand, "now this is very important" may help them to remember what follows.

3. Give reasons for key advice. Tell **why** it is necessary to continue medication usage, such as using an antibiotic even though symptoms have disappeared. Sophisticated patients need to understand the reasons behind what you and the physician are instructing them.

4. Give definite, concrete, explicit instructions. Any information that patients can mentally picture is more easily remembered. Use visual aids, photographs, or demonstrations. When patients are given specific, easy-to-understand instructions, they tend to regard this advice as more important than if it is given in general terms.

5. Present key information at the beginning or end of the interaction. Experience has shown that patients concentrate on the initial information given and remember best the last items discussed.

6. Supplement the spoken word with written instructions. By so doing, you can pare down face-to-face consultations to essentials and at the same time provide patients with information to refer to as needed. Selecting the appropriate written information is crucial, since the quality and quantity of material are varied. The material must be comprehensive, yet presented in an interesting format.

7. Finally, end the encounter by giving patients the opportunity to provide feedback about what they learned. Ask patients to restate critical points of information to check for accuracy. This type of approach prevents having the process become strictly one-way communication.

Techniques to Improve Patient Behavior

Attempting to change patient behavior related to the wise use of medications is a very complex process, and, again, it is beyond the scope of this textbook to describe the various behavioral interventions that appear to be effective in improving patient compliance. Pharmacists can certainly learn from the experience of public health educators, since they have developed practical, proven techniques to change social behaviors such as wearing seatbelts, recycling glass and newspaper, exercising, reducing cholesterol intake, and stopping smoking. The reader is also referred to the work of pharmacists and researchers who have established effective medication adherence programs. For example, Armstrong and Newberg (1994) describe several strategies to enhance pharmaceutical care. Prochaska and Velicer (1997) have successfully applied elements of the Transtheoretical Model to improve patient adherence to medication regimens. Studies involving the Health Belief Model (Ried and Christensen, 1988; Richardson et al, 1993) and Self Efficacy (Johnson, 1996; Taal et al, 1993) have also provided insight into how pharmacists can work with patients on improving their therapeutic outcomes.

Most of the previous strategies rely on effective patient–pharmacist communication. These strategies are effective only if used in a caring environment by pharmacists with empathetic communication skills. Application of elements of these models is certainly enhanced by strong communication skills. You should consider the following points when designing your interventions to enhance adherence (Box 9.2):

1. Integrate new behaviors with current behaviors. It is hard for someone to establish new behaviors unless he or she is tied to existing behaviors. One approach that appears to be effective is linking new behaviors (taking a medication) to a set of typical behaviors, such as brushing teeth in the morning or going to bed, preparing dinner, or dressing for work in the morning. Other strategies include setting wristwatches or other alarms, posting reminder notes in obvious places, and storing medications where they will be seen at the time that they are to be taken.

2. Provide appropriate aids. Individualized medication packaging for daily or weekly doses seems to work for some patients (Smith, 1989). Digital timepieces installed in some vial caps help patients monitor when medications are taken (McKenney et al, 1992).

3. Suggest ways to self-monitor. One simple way to help patients is to suggest that they use a medication diary or calendar on which to record their medication use. In addition, seeing differences in body function can be a strong reinforcement regarding their medications. Thus, patients can monitor their response to treatment, such as taking their own blood pressure or testing their blood glucose levels.

4. Monitor medication use. With chronic care medications, you should monitor adherence frequently and assess patient perception of effectiveness and problems encountered. You should review prescription records for potential problems, such as pat-

---

Box 9.2 STRATEGIES TO ENHANCE ADHERENCE TO
MEDICATION REGIMENS

- Integrate new behaviors into patient lifestyle.
- Provide or suggest compliance or reminder aids.
- Suggest patient self-monitoring.
- Monitor use on an ongoing basis.
- Refer patients when necessary.

terns of late refills. Refill-reminder software systems are available to generate reports and to implement reminder systems, such as creating reminder postcards when refills are due. Many pharmacists call patients to see how they are doing after they start on a new prescription.

5. In some cases, you may want to refer patients to appropriate social service agencies, such as government programs for low-income patients. Barriers to proper adherence can include the inability of the patient to obtain needed medications.

SUMMARY

Successful patient adherence has both knowledge and behavioral components. In other words, patients must not only know key points of information about their medication but must also perform specific behaviors (i.e., taking medication at a certain time, using an inhaler correctly) to optimize therapeutic outcomes. Adherence to medication regimens can be improved by enhancing patient understanding about the medication and by facilitating the patient's ability to take the medication correctly. Thus, you must assess patient knowledge about medication and educate patients regarding essential information. You must also assess patient medication-taking behavior and provide strategies to enhance these behaviors.

Communication to achieve better outcomes is often complex. Many people find sharing private matters difficult, and therefore they resist developing a relationship in which teamwork is the goal. If patients feel no rapport with their pharmacist, two-way communication will be diminished and the patient's care ultimately suffers. Assessing patient understanding as part of the patient counseling process can be ineffective if misperceptions exist about patient attitudes and assumptions about taking prescribed medication. To help patients become more self-directed at taking their medications, you first must develop feedback that allows you to understand what they understand and believe about their medications as well as how they are actually using the medications. Only then can you assess nonadherent behavior and make suggestions to improve medication use.

REVIEW QUESTIONS

1. What is a most likely reason for a pharmacist's inability to help patients take medication as prescribed?
2. What false assumptions do pharmacists often make that cloud otherwise clear communication?

3. What are several techniques that assist a pharmacist in assessing a patient's knowledge about medication?

4. Can you describe at least five techniques that help you "partner" with a patient to motivate him or her into compliance with therapy?

5. Describe several special communication techniques that can be used to effectively improve a pharmacist–patient encounter.

References

Armstrong EP, Newberg DA. Discussing pharmaceutical care on a grass-roots basis. *Journal of the American Pharmaceutical Association* NS34: 38–47, 1994.

Ell KO. Coping with serious illness. *International Journal of Psychiatric Medicine* 15:335–356, 1986.

Hepler CD, Strand LM. Opportunities and responsibilities in pharmaceutical care. *American Journal of Hospital Pharmacy* 47: 533–543, 1990.

Hill MN. Strategies for patient education. *Clinical and Experimental Hypertension* A11(5–6), 1989.

Institute of Medicine. *Crossing the Quality Chasm: A New Health System for the 21st Century.* Washington, DC, 2001.

Johnson JA. Self-efficacy theory as a framework for community pharmacy-based diabetes education programs. *The Diabetes Educator* 22:237–241, 1996.

Lasagna L. Noncompliance data and clinical outcomes. *Drug Topics Supplement* Montvale, NJ, 1992.

Ley P. Doctor-patient relationships. *Journal of Hypertension* 3:51–55, 1985.

McKenney JM. Pharmacists' guidelines for fostering compliance among patients with asymptomatic conditions requiring chronic therapy. *NARD Journal* (Special Supplement) 35–40, June 1990.

McKenney JM, Munroe WP, Wright JT, Jr. Impact of an electronic medication compliance aid on long-term blood pressure control. *Journal of Clinical Pharmacology* 32:277–283, 1992.

Prochaska JO, Velicer WF. The Transtheoretical Model of health behavior change. *American Journal of Health Promotion* 12: 38–48. 1997.

Richardson MA, Simons-Morton B, Annegers JF. Effect of perceived barriers on compliance with antihypertensive medication. *Health Education Quarterly* 20:489–503, 1993.

Ried LD, Christensen DB. A psychosocial perspective in the explanation of patients' drug-taking behavior. *Social Science & Medicine* 27: 277–285, 1988.

Smith DL. Compliance packaging: a powerful marketing tool. *Trends and Forecasts.* National Pharmaceutical Council 2:3, 1989.

Svarstad BL. Patient-practitioner relationships and compliance with prescribed medical regiments. In Aiken LH, Mechanic D, eds. *Application of Social Sciences to Clinical Medicine on Health Policy.* New Brunswick NJ: Rutgers, University Press, 1986: 438–459.

Taal E, Rasker JJ, Seydel ER, Wiegman O. Health status, adherence with health recommendations, self-efficacy and social support in patients with rheumatoid arthritis. *Patient Education and Counseling* 20:63–76, 1993.

Suggested Readings

Coons SJ, Sheahan SL, Martin SS, et al. Predictors of medication noncompliance in a sample of older adults. *Clinical Therapeutics* 16: 1, 1994.

Fincham JE, Wertheimer AI. Using the Health Belief Model to predict initial drug therapy default. *Social Science & Medicine* 20: 101–105, 1985.

Leibowitz K. Improving your patient counseling skills. *American Pharmacy* N533: 65–69, 1993.

Morris LS, Schulz RM. Medication compliance: the patient's perspective. *Clinical Therapeutics* 15:3, 1993.

Morris LS, Schulz RM. Patient compliance—an overview. *Journal of Clinical Pharmacology and Therapeutics* 17: 283–295, 1992.

Nagasawa M, Smith MC, Barnes JH, Fincham SE. Meta-analysis of correlates of diabetes patients' compliance with prescribed medications. *The Diabetes Educator* 16:192–200, 1991.

Smith MC. The cost of noncompliance and the capacity of improved compliance to reduce health care expenditures. In *National Pharmaceutical Council: A Symposium*. Washington, DC, 1985.

Chapter 10

Communication with Special Patients

▨ OVERVIEW

Applying communication skills to pharmacy practice situations is not always easy. It can be especially difficult in situations in which patients have special communication needs. These situations require special sensitivities and unique strategies to ensure effective communication. This chapter addresses the skills needed to deal with older adults, persons with hearing, sight, or literacy deficiencies, terminally ill patients, patients with AIDS, patients with mental health problems, and persons taking care of patients ("caregivers").

Introduction

Communication in pharmacy practice is frequently hindered by specific challenges presented by unique groups of patients. This chapter discusses specific communication barriers involving a variety of situations. Different strategies are also outlined to assist you in identifying and dealing with these special communication needs.

Before discussing the unique communication challenges of these special patient groups, one caveat that applies to most situations must be offered: if you sense that a person has a unique problem, you should check your perception of that problem (see Chapter 3). An example is how we often treat the elderly. Although some elderly patients may appear to be frail, they may not be forgetful or hearing-impaired. However, we make certain assumptions based on our perceptions of the elderly as a group of patients. Thus, we may start shouting at them or talking slower. The key is to assess how they are responding to our educational efforts. We should watch for nonverbal clues to see if they are leaning toward us or if they have a confused look. Asking open-ended questions can also provide feedback about the patient's ability to communicate. Not checking initial impressions could lead to some potentially embarrassing situations both for patients and for us. We should try to avoid stereotyping individuals and make sure to check our perceptions.

Older Adults

Several factors make it imperative for pharmacists to be sensitive to interactions involving older adults. The number of elderly in our society is increasing, and the elderly consume a disproportionate amount of prescription and nonprescription medications compared with other age groups. Elderly men and women present special opportunities for pharmacists because they account for 30% of all prescription medication taken in the United States and 40% of all OTC medication. As a group, two out of three elderly people take at least one medication daily. Thus, this growing segment of the population is in need of our patient counseling services. Unfortunately, the aging process sometimes affects certain elements of the communication process in some older adults. These potential communication problems are discussed below. In addition, several of the communication impairments such as hearing loss and aphasia have special implications in elderly populations. These impairments are discussed later in the chapter.

Learning

In certain individuals, the aging process affects the learning process, but not the ability to learn. Some older adults learn at a slower rate than younger persons. They have the ability to learn, but they process information at a different rate. Thus, the rate of speech and the amount of information presented at one time must meet the individual's ability to comprehend the material. In addition, short-term memory, recall, and attention span may be diminished in some elderly patients. The ability to process new and innovative solutions to problems might also be slower in some older adults. Thus, attempts to change behaviors should be structured gradually and should build on past experiences. A good approach with some older adults is to set reasonable short-term goals, approach long-term goals in stages, and break down learning tasks into smaller components. Another important step is to encourage feedback from patients as to whether they received your intended message by tactfully asking them to repeat instructions and other information and by watching their nonverbal responses. When given the opportunity to learn at their own speed, most elderly people can learn as well as younger adults.

Value and Perceptual Differences

Potential communication barriers between you and older patients may be attributable to the generation gap. Some older adults may perceive things differently from those in different age groups, since people typically adhere to values learned and accepted in their younger years. Thus, some older adults may have different beliefs and perceptions about health care in general and about drugs and pharmacists specifically. Some behaviors, such as hoarding and sharing medication, may seem inappropriate to you, but such actions may make sense to someone who grew up in the 1930s during the Depression. You should be aware of situations in which you may be reacting to their different values and belief systems rather than to the patients themselves.

The image of the pharmacist is also important. Older patients may expect a well-groomed, clean-shaven, professional-looking male practitioner to serve them. If you do not meet these expectations, they may be somewhat reluctant to interact with you initially. Their perception of authority may also influence how they interact with you. Some older adults grew up respecting the authority of physicians and pharmacists and prefer a more directed approach to receiving health care. Thus, they may be receptive to being told what to do. On the other hand, other patients may want to be more independent and may feel a need to assert themselves. So they may be somewhat more demanding, may want additional information, or may want more input into the medication decision-making process. Thus, it is important to assess which approach seems to work for each patient.

Psychosocial Factors

Several psychosocial factors may influence your relationship with older adults. First, some older adults may be experiencing a significant amount of loss compared with people of other age groups. For example, their friends may be dying at an increased rate; they may have retired from their jobs; or they may have had to slow down or cease certain activities owing to the aging process. All these situations involve loss

Review Case 10.1

Nellie Curtis, age 83, has been a member of a large managed-care plan since its inception in 1975. She became a member as part of her husband's employee benefits package when his employer converted shortly after his retirement. She has always had her prescriptions filled at the clinic pharmacy run by the HMO. On this occasion she enters the pharmacy to pick up refills for two of her medications, a diuretic and a digitalis glycoside. Marcus, the pharmacist, greets Nellie:

> **Marcus:** *Hello Nellie! I bet you are having a good day today.*
>
> **Nellie:** *Not really, but why are you so sure?*
>
> **Marcus:** *Because with all this rain we've been having it's gotta be good for the crops and making the grass green.*
>
> **Nellie:** *Well I guess so.*
>
> **Marcus:** *Here are your medicines. Let's see, you take one of each once a day, except the little white one is every other day. Right?*
>
> **Nellie:** *Yup, I think you've got it.*
>
> **Marcus:** *You have been on this stuff a long time, haven't you?*
>
> **Nellie:** *Yup, 'bout a decade.*
>
> **Marcus:** *You're not having any problems with them, are you?*
>
> **Nellie:** *Well, I mustn't be, I'm still around aren't I? Say, why all the questions?*
>
> **Marcus:** *It's our new policy to talk to people. There is a law that says we need to talk more to customers.*
>
> **Nellie:** *It's about time!*
>
> **Marcus:** *Well Nellie, y'all have a good one.*

How could have Marcus better prepared this elderly patient for a counseling encounter?

How should he have established a more respectful relationship?

How could have Marcus assessed and responded to any of Nellie's needs related to sight, hearing, or memory loss?

What simple sentences could Marcus have used to assure Nellie's understanding of how and why she takes her medicines?

Some of Marcus' comments appeared to be leading, restrictive, and judgmental in nature. Rewrite Marcus' dialogue to let Nellie respond with items that are important to her.

and subsequent grieving. Thus, their reaction to certain medical situations, such as ignoring your directions or complaining about the price of their medications, may be responses to fear of their diseases, of becoming even less active, or of dying. They may deny the situation or become angry at you or other health care providers. They may also turn to self-diagnosis and self-treatment or to the use of other people's medications.

Communication Impairments

Box 10.1 summarizes patient impairments to communication.

Vision

Pharmacists in a variety of practice settings work with patients with visual impairments. So be prepared to offer alternative forms of patient counseling to deal with these impairments. If you work with elderly patients, you need to realize that the aging process may affect the visual process. Written messages for persons with visual deficiencies should be in large print and on pastel-colored paper rather than on white paper. Many times visual acuity is not as sharp, and sensitivity to color is decreased. In some older patients, more light is needed to stimulate the receptors in the eye. Thus, when using written information, make sure you have enough light.

Hearing

Three general types of physical hearing impairment (conductive, sensorineural, and central) can occur singly or in combination with one another. Conductive hearing impairment results when something blocks the conduction of sound into the ear's sensory nerve centers. Sensorineural impairment occurs when the problem is situated in the sensory center of the inner ear. Central hearing impairment occurs when the nerve centers within the brain are affected. A hearing aid is helpful for people with conductive hearing problems, less effective for those with sensorineural impairment, and ineffective for those with

---

Box 10.1 POSSIBLE PATIENT IMPAIRMENTS

- Vision
- Hearing
- Speech
- Aphasia

central loss. Because the hearing aid only makes the sound louder, it is not as helpful in patients who cannot distinguish sounds easily and may actually make some situations worse. Hearing deficiencies can also be caused by a variety of factors, including birth defects, injuries, and chronic exposure to loud noises.

Aging may also affect the hearing process. Auditory loss in various degrees of severity is seen in more than 50% of all older adults. The hearing loss associated with the aging process is called *presbycusis.* Unfortunately, this condition may lead individuals to withdraw socially and psychologically or, in extreme cases, may lead others to label them as senile or forgetful. Many older adults describe their hearing impairment as being able to hear what others are saying, but not being able to understand what is being said. They can hear words, but they cannot put them together clearly. Other types of hearing loss seen in some older adults are related to diminished response to high-frequency sounds. In some older adults, sensitivity to sound is decreased, and the volume must be increased to stimulate the receptors.

Many individuals with hearing deficiencies, including some older adults, rely on speech-reading (watching the lips, facial expressions, and gestures) to enhance their communication ability. Speech-reading is more than just lip-reading. It involves receiving visual cues from facial expressions, body postures, and gestures as well as lip movements. Research has shown that everyone develops some speech-reading skill and that the hearing-impaired need to develop that skill much further. Development of this skill is further hindered if sight is impaired as well, as in some older adults. For speech-reading to be most effective, you should position patients directly in front of you and have a light shining on your lips and face when communicating.

To improve communication with hearing-impaired patients, try to position yourself about 3 to 6 feet away; never speak directly into the patient's ear because this may distort the message. Wait until the patient can see you before speaking; position yourself on the side of patient's strongest ear; and, if necessary, touch the patient on the arm. If your message does not appear to be getting through, you should not keep repeating the same statement, but rephrase it in shorter, simpler sentences. Many pharmacists have learned sign language to assist hearing-impaired patients.

Other types of hearing loss seen in some older adults are related to the actual hearing process. Response to high-frequency sounds is usually diminished before the response to lower sounds. Thus, using a lower tone of voice may help some older adults. In some older persons, sensitivity to sound is decreased, and increased volume can assist in hearing. It is also important to slow your rate of speech somewhat so that the person can differentiate the words. Remember not to shout when speaking, since shouting may offend some people. Talking in a somewhat higher volume may be necessary, but more likely a slower rate of speech will help most individuals. Finally, be aware of environmental barriers, such as loud background noises or dimly lit counseling areas, which make communication difficult for the hearing-impaired.

Speech

In pharmacy practice, you may need to interact with people who have some type of speech impairment. Speech deficiencies can be caused by a variety of factors, such as birth defects, injuries, or illnesses. A common speech deficiency is *dysarthria*, or interference with normal control of the speech mechanism. Diseases, such as Parkinson's disease, multiple sclerosis, and bulbar palsy, as well as strokes and accidents, can cause dysarthria. In dysarthria, speech may be slurred or otherwise difficult to understand because of lack of ability to produce speech sounds correctly, maintain good breath control, or coordinate the movements of the lips, tongue, palate, and larynx. Many of these patients can be helped by certain medications or by therapy from a trained speech pathologist.

Another common speech problem results from the removal of the larynx secondary to throat cancer or other conditions. Such individuals can usually learn to speak again either by learning esophageal speech or by using an electronic device. However, you must be sensitive to these patients, since they sound "different." Many people realize they sound different and that they may make other people feel uncomfortable. Thus, they may shy away from interacting with others.

To overcome speech barriers, many patients write notes to their pharmacist or use sign language as a means of communicating. Some pharmacists have responded to this need by providing writing pads for patients and even by learning how to sign along with the patient.

Aphasia

A group of patients with related speech difficulties are those who suffer from aphasia after a stroke or another adverse event. *Aphasia* is a complex problem, which may result, to varying degrees, in the reduced ability to understand what others are saying and to express oneself. Some patients may have no speech, whereas others may have only mild difficulties in recalling names or words. Others may have problems putting words in their proper order in a sentence. Speech may be limited to short phrases or single words; or, smaller words are left out so that the sentence reads like a telegram. The ability to understand oral directions, to read, to write, and to deal with numbers may also be disturbed. Fortunately for some patients, their communication ability can be improved after extensive therapy. However, improvements are often seen in small increments.

Aphasic patients usually have normal hearing acuity; shouting at them will not help. Their problems are due to lack of comprehension; they are not hard of hearing, stubborn, or inattentive. Until you are aware of the extent of language impairment, avoid complex conversations. You need to be patient with these individuals when discussing their medications. Many times, they get frustrated with their situation because they know what they want to say but cannot say it. Also, it takes longer to communicate with them, since they may hear the word but may not immediately recall the meaning of it. Patience is also needed, since you may be tempted to fill in the word or phrase for aphasic patients. It is best to let them try to communicate. If they are unsuccessful after a few attempts, help them by supplying a few words in multiple-choice fashion and let them select the word they desire. Aphasic patients often feel isolated and may withdraw from social interactions. Thus, they should be encouraged to interact with other people. Most appreciate being included in a conversation even if only to listen.

Some aphasic patients have difficulty reading. The difficulty is not one of visual acuity but rather of comprehending written language. Some have severe dyslexia and cannot read at all; others can read single words with comprehension but cannot read sentences. Patients with dyslexia may not be able to write notes to you. Dyslexia is not a physical disability but rather the inability to recall or form conventional written symbols.

Many aphasic patients retain certain automatic responses and may appear to be able to communicate very well. They may be able to count to 10 but not to count 4 items placed in front of them. They can name the days of the week, but not tell you that Tuesday comes before Thursday. They may be able to function effectively only in repetitive situations. Usually, their automatic speech skills are within socially acceptable limits, but sometimes patients utter profanities that may embarrass both listeners and patients themselves. Patients are not displaying anger or other displeasures when they curse, but rather are using automatic speech and are unable to inhibit these responses. You will probably be challenged when counseling aphasic patients and getting feedback may be difficult, but you should at least make an attempt, since they may benefit from the experience. Many times it is best to counsel other people who are caring for aphasic patients, but do not exclude patients from this experience.

Terminally Ill Patients

Most individuals, including pharmacists, find it somewhat difficult to interact with terminally ill patients. People typically feel uncomfortable discussing the topic of death and are uncertain about what to say; they do not want to say the "wrong'" thing or upset patients. Yet, most terminally ill patients need supportive relationships from family members, friends, and pharmacists.

Pharmacists are becoming increasingly important in the care of terminally ill patients owing to the complex nature of cancer therapy and pain management and to their increased involvement on oncology teams in hospitals and other institutions. By the same token, more community-based pharmacists are getting involved because of the de-institutionalization of cancer treatment and the evolution of home health care as a popular option for many patients. More important, pharmacists may be the only health professionals in their community who are readily accessible to patients and families. Thus, you should be ready, professionally and emotionally, to interact with these patients.

The following communication strategies should be used when working with terminally ill patients. Many of these approaches are too complex to be discussed in detail here but are listed in the recommended readings at the end of this chapter (Beardsley et al, 1977; Feifel, 1977; Kubler-Ross, 1969). Most strategies require "meeting the patients where they are" in relation to their understanding of their condition and their stage of adjustment. For example, a patient may be denying the existence of his illness, or he may be angry or depressed about his situation. You would approach these two situations differently. The key is to ask open-ended questions, such as "how are you doing today?" or "how are things going?" to determine patient willingness to discuss the situation with you. You should not assume that patients do not want to talk about it. Even if patients do not respond initially, they at least realize that you are willing to talk and may open up at a later time.

Before interacting with terminally ill patients, be aware of your own feelings about death and about interacting with terminally ill patients. Do you typically avoid conversations with these patients? Do they remind you of someone close to you who struggles with a terminal illness? Being aware of your feelings will help you assist these patients. You should realize that you can handle some situations yourself, whereas other cases should be referred to others for assistance. Many pharmacists have found that just being honest about their feelings improves their interaction with terminally ill patients. Just by saying "I don't know what to say right now. Tell me how I can help you?" or "I feel so helpless. Is there anything I can do for you?" seems to communicate concern for patients and gives them a chance to share their concerns as well. As in any type of patient interaction, the degree of involvement depends on your relationship with the patient. You will be more open with some patients than with others. It is also important to implicitly or explicitly set limits on what you can do for the patient. You must communicate your concern without raising patient expectations that you can assist in all areas of the patient's life, such as providing financial advice or preparing a will.

Many terminally ill patients realize they make other people feel uncomfortable. Thus, they tend to avoid certain interactions. However, if you can express your uneasiness or your frustration about not knowing how to help them at the same time that you express your concern for them, patients will typically feel more at ease and more willing to express their own feelings.

You may also come in contact with family members who will probably have special needs themselves. Research has shown that family members go through the same type of stages that dying patients go through, and thus they need support and often drug therapy (Kubler-Ross, 1969). You may be called on to be a good listener to lend support to the family members.

In summary, communicating with terminally ill patients and their families is extremely important. You should not avoid talking with them unless you sense that they do not want to talk about their illness. Not interacting with them only contributes further to their isolation and may reaffirm the idea that talking about death is uncomfortable.

Patients with AIDS

As a pharmacist, you will probably be working with patients who have a variety of health issues revolving around acquired immune deficiency syndrome (AIDS). Not only are these patients dealing with potentially life-threatening diseases, they are also dealing with the social stigmas that often accompany their condition. The key is not to treat them as being "different" from your other patients. Typically, they do have a unique set of needs that need to be recognized and addressed. Many of the issues discussed in the terminally ill section apply to AIDS patients, since AIDS can be a terminal disease. However, many patients are living much longer life spans since the advent of highly active antiretroviral therapy. Therefore, health professionals must adjust their thinking and come to perceive HIV infection as a chronic condition rather than a terminal disease. In any case, you should use some of the strategies outlined in the previous text, such as using open-ended questions to determine patient receptivity to interaction.

Patients with AIDS have special needs that should be considered. For example, many patients do not have an adequate support system,

REVIEW CASE 10.2

Mary Jane Marvel is a 22-year-old college senior. For the past semester, she has had a nagging vaginal infection. She recently volunteered to give blood at a local Red Cross chapter, but unfortunately she tested positive for HIV during the blood screening process. She became scared and angry and went to a doctor, where she was still too confused to talk about the HIV test but did talk about the nagging vaginal infection. The doctor gave her a prescription for a common antifungal/yeast agent. She approaches the campus health pharmacy with trepidation and stands off to one side while Stephanie, the pharmacist, fills the prescription. Stephanie notices Mary Jane's behavior and leaves the prescription counter to talk with her.

> **Stephanie:** *Hello Miss Marvel, I am Stephanie Gonzales, and as the pharmacist who filled your prescription, I would like to talk to you a little bit about it. Is this okay?*

> **Mary Jane:** *Sure, why not (said nervously).*

> **Stephanie:** *I was watching you a moment ago and you seem very distressed.*

> **Mary Jane:** *How would you feel if you had to stick that stuff inside you? Besides, why should I confide in you?*

> **Stephanie:** *I may be able to help by providing information about your treatment.*

> **Mary Jane:** *Well since you zeroed in on my feelings so accurately, I guess I must tell someone before I burst.*

> **Stephanie:** *I do respect your trust and confidence, but before we talk, let's step over here to a more private area.*

> **Mary Jane:** *I failed an HIV test and I am scared I am going to die.*

Analyze Stephanie's ability to take Mary Jane into her confidence.

Discuss the barriers Stephanie may have to interacting with an HIV patient.

What nonverbal behavior could Stephanie display that indicates she is ready to listen?

Discuss the following attributes to evaluate Stephanie's approach as an active listener:

> Did she listen to understand?

> Did she empathize to show she cared?

> Did she hold back arguments so as not to appear judgmental?

> Did she ask questions to clarify feelings and understanding?

since relationships with family and friends are somewhat strained because of the social stigma. You may be asked to be part of the patient's support system or called on to refer the patient to an appropriate source of support. You may need to supply additional triage or problem-solving support, since others are not providing it.

Many patients have trouble dealing with their own identity as the disease progresses. In many cases, dealing with AIDS has a physical component (i.e., weight loss, lack of energy), but also psychological and sociological aspects (i.e., becoming more dependent on others, fear of dying, fear of pain). People with AIDS are wrestling with a lot of issues and may need some assistance sorting things out.

Patients must also deal with misinformation and inaccurate perceptions about AIDS. People around them may not understand the various aspects of the disease or its treatment. It is hoped that pharmacists are not included in this misinformed group. We must keep up with the latest literature, since we know that many AIDS patients monitor what is being researched. You must determine what your role should be in assisting these patients. You may or may not feel comfortable becoming a close member of patient support networks or taking an active role in ensuring that patient needs are met beyond your professional responsibility to provide pharmaceutical care services. The key is to identify what the patient's needs are and what services you can provide or referrals you can make to best meet these needs.

Patients with Mental Health Problems

Many pharmacists admit that they have difficulty in communicating with another group of patients: those with mental health disorders. By the same token, many mental health patients may be reluctant to interact with other individuals. Some pharmacists feel that they do not know what to say to mental health patients. They are afraid to say the wrong thing or something that might cause an emotional outburst by the patient in the pharmacy. Some pharmacists are also unsure of how much information to provide to such patients about their condition and treatment. Many times it is unclear what patients already understand about their condition and what their physicians have told them. Once again, open-ended questions are good tools to use to determine the level of patient understanding before you counsel them about their medications. Examples include, "What has the doctor told you about this medication?" or "This drug can be used for different things. What has your physician said?" Asking open-ended questions also helps you determine patient cognitive functioning. That is, are they able to comprehend what you are saying, and can they articulate their concerns to you? If not, you may have to communicate through a caregiver or someone else.

Some pharmacists may also be reluctant to distribute written information to patients receiving psychotropic medications for fear that patients may misinterpret the information. Another related concern is that many psychotropic medications, such as imipramine for bed-wetting and diazepam for muscle spasms, are used for non–mental health disorders. Thus, the written material may not be relevant to the patient's condition and may only cause alarm. It is important that you carefully screen all materials for their relevance to the individual patient before distribution and that you make an attempt to verbally reinforce the information to ensure a better understanding by the patient.

Pharmacists interacting with patients with mental disorders must address a more fundamental ethical issue: should patients with mental disorders be allowed the same level of information regarding their drug treatment and the same type of informed consent as patients with nonpsychiatric disorders? Does the uniqueness of having a mental illness versus a physical illness preclude these patients from knowing more about the effects (both positive and negative) of their drugs? Do we withhold certain information that would be given to a nonpsychiatric patient? Obviously, each situation must be evaluated individually, and many times in consultation with the patient's physician. However, the issue is raised here because the way you deal with these questions affects how you communicate with mental health patients. In some situations, trusting relationships may develop among patients, mental health practitioners, and pharmacists. In these cases, pharmacists can be key members of the patient's care management team.

REVIEW CASE 10.3

A patient who looks somewhat depressed approaches the prescription counter.

> "Boy, I can't believe what is happening to me. I went to the doctor because I was feeling kind of low. She gave me a prescription for Ambien (zolpidem). It certainly helps me sleep, but I still feel depressed. Did you ever wonder if life was worth the hassle?"

How would you respond to this person?

What special needs does this patient seem to have?

What is your role in this situation?

Unfortunately, certain stereotypes about mental illness and patients with these disorders tend to inhibit communication. People in general, as well as many pharmacists, have certain stigmas and misconceptions about mental illness. We tend to categorize people based on images from the media or from beliefs we have formed about how "crazy" people act. Our reluctance is also reinforced by the fact that some patients indeed act "different." They may have awkward body and facial movements (possibly owing to their medications). Some are chronic cigarette smokers and have poor hygienic habits. They may make what we consider to be bizarre statements. They may not establish good eye contact, which may make us even more uncomfortable.

Patients with mental illness may be reluctant to interact with pharmacists for a variety of reasons. First, they may have a poor self-concept and may be insecure about interacting with others. They may also realize that they have a condition that makes other people uncomfortable. Thus, this societal stigma about mental illness makes them avoid social interactions. In some cases, patients may be paranoid about dealing with other people, especially health care professionals. Thus, your attempts to communicate may find initial patient resistance. Patients with mental illness typically need multiple contacts to establish trusting relationships. However, you should realize that this may never happen and that your interactions may always be "different" compared with your relationships with other patients. These differences should be handled the same way that you deal with other unique individuals discussed in previous sections. Differences should not stop you from trying to interact with these special patients. However, the potential communication problems may require you to be innovative in developing strategies to overcome them.

Patients with Low Health Literacy

Low health literacy is a pervasive problem that impedes the ability of many patients to understand information we provide them about their medications. Health literacy is the ability to "read, understand and act on healthcare information." (AMA, 1999). To illustrate the extent of the problem, one study found that 42% of patients could not read and comprehend directions for administering a medication on an empty stomach (Williams et al, 1995). Persons with limited ability to read and comprehend information are frequently embarrassed and fail to disclose this fact to health care providers. At the same time, health care professionals are largely unaware of the extent of the problem in society and in their own population of patients. Providers also fail to assess patients' understanding of written information provided to them. Some research has found that providing pictures with accompanying simple written instructions can improve comprehension of key medication instructions, such as the appropriate timing of doses (Morrow et al, 1998). The *United States Pharmacopeia* (USP) has developed 81 pictograms that illustrate common medication instructions and precautions. These graphic images can be downloaded from the USP website (www.usp.org) and used by health care professionals to supplement written instructions for low literate or non–English-speaking patients. In addition, the American Medical Association Foundation has produced a Health Literacy Introductory Kit for health care providers describing the scope of the health literacy problem and suggesting ways to overcome barriers to communicating with low-literacy patients (www.ama-assn.org).

Caregivers

Several special communication problems arise when pharmacists must interact with patient caregivers rather than with the patients themselves. Caregivers can be people who take care of older adults with chronic conditions, parents who take care of children during acute illnesses, family members, friends or hired assistants. In general, the number of these caregivers will probably increase in the future, since there has been an increased effort to shift patient care from hospitals to home care. Dealing with caregivers takes a set of specific strategies, since you cannot communicate directly with patients and thus cannot determine whether they received your intended message. It is also difficult to assess patient adherence with medication regimens and to offer support and encouragement to patients regarding their medication treatment.

When dealing with caregivers, certain areas should be addressed. First, caregivers need to understand the patient's condition and treatment and how to communicate specific instructions to the patient. Caregivers must also understand how to monitor patient therapeutic response to a specific medication, how to monitor for adverse drug events, and how to report any suspicious events. They should be instructed on the importance of good nutrition and fluid intake for certain types of patients. They must be reminded about the refill status of medications and when the physicians need to be contacted. Caregivers should be encouraged to contact you if they have any questions or if the patient has specific questions.

Written information about the medication is essential, since the message should be delivered to patients. A follow-up phone call to patients may also be necessary to make sure that messages were received and to reinforce key points regarding drug therapy. Many pharmacists use medication reminder systems (i.e., drug calendars, weekly medication containers) to help caregivers keep track of medications.

REVIEW CASE 10.4

Mrs. Hope is 70 years old and takes care of her husband John who is also 70. John is confined at home because of his Alzheimer's condition. Mrs. Hope has taken John to a physician for a check-up and now meets Rebecca Dorsey, the pharmacist, in the outpatient clinic pharmacy in the hospital, where the physician holds privileges.

Rebecca: Good morning, Mrs. Hope. How are you today?

Mrs. Hope: I'm ok, but I'm concerned about these new prescriptions. One is for me, the other is for my husband John.

Rebecca: May I please read them?

Mrs. Hope: Yes, go ahead.

Rebecca: Which one concerns you?

Mrs. Hope: They both do. With the one for John, I was never told why it was prescribed. The second one for me is something I've never had before.

Rebecca: Well, John's prescription is for a diuretic. That means it's a water pill, and it works to remove extra fluid from inside the body. Your prescription is what we call a nonsteroidal anti-inflammatory drug. It's used to reduce the inflammation and pain associated with conditions like arthritis.

Mrs. Hope: But, John has Alzheimer's and I do not have arthritis. The doctor is new and has only seen us once. Why would he prescribe such stuff?

Mrs. Hope is obviously the caregiver and, as such, requires special attention. What could she be feeling? What open-ended questions could Rebecca have used to initiate the conversation and prevent making false assumptions? What false assumptions contributed to Rebecca's ineffectiveness? What could Rebecca have done to ensure that both patients follow the medication regimens? What could Rebecca have done or said to encourage and support Mrs. Hope in the care of her husband?

In addition, you should develop a special sensitivity to caregivers and should not merely view them as someone picking up the medication. Many times, caregivers have special needs themselves. They may be under a lot of stress trying to care for the patient at home. They may have careers and other activities outside the home and may be financially strained as well. Serious depression has been found in almost one-fourth of the individuals caring for the home-bound elderly. In some situations, the caregivers may be patients themselves with their own medical problems. It is interesting to note that one of the fastest-growing segments of our population is the group of people over 65 with parents in their 80s and 90s (Elderhealth, 1986). Thus, two generations of patients with health problems may be living in the same home.

You should also respond empathetically to caregivers and try to understand some of their personal problems. As mentioned earlier, pharmacists are often the most accessible health care professionals in the community and may be the only consistent contact caregivers have with the health care network. You should be aware of the caregiver's nonverbal messages and must not be afraid to ask, "What is on your mind?" You should also be aware of the different support groups in the community that could assist caregivers, such as local hospice organizations for terminally ill patients at home or respite care services to ease caregiver burden. You should realize that dealing with a terminal illness or other devastating disease may reduce family members' ability to communicate with each other and health care providers. Caregivers have so much stress in their daily lives that it is difficult for them to express their exact needs.

SUMMARY

You will always be challenged by situations needing special attention as a pharmacist. Although the groups discussed in this chapter do not represent the entire universe of patients with special communication needs, they do reflect groups that deserve special consideration in pharmacy practice. The following chapter addresses another special group of patients—children who are dealing with health issues. With all patients, pharmacists need to first recognize patients with special communication needs and then develop effective strategies to overcome these specific barriers to the communication process as outlined above.

REVIEW QUESTIONS

1. What impact does aging have on learning, memory, and recall?
2. Is there such a thing as a generation gap when counseling patients? If so, explain.
3. What is aphasia, and how can you communicate with a patient who has it?
4. Describe your feelings about the terminally ill and how you could best communicate with them.
5. What are some of the special communication problems that arise from interactions with caregivers?

References

AMA Ad Hoc Committee on Health Literacy. Health Literacy: Report of the Council on Scientific Affairs. *JAMA* 281: 552–557, 1999.

Beardsley RS, Johnson CA, Benson SB. Pharmacist interaction with the terminally ill patient. *Journal of the American Pharmaceutical Association* NS17: 750–752, 1977.

Elderhealth. Consumer drug education program. Maryland Pharm 62:4, 1986.

Feifel H. *New Meanings of Death.* New York: McGraw-Hill, 1977.

Kubler-Ross E. *On Death and Dying.* New York: Macmillan, 1969.

Morrow DG, Hier CM, Menard WE, Leirer VO. Icons improve older and younger adults' comprehension of medication information. *Journal of Gerontology* 53: P240–P254, 1998.

Williams MU, Parker RM, Baker DW et al. Inadequate functional health literacy among patients at two public hospitals. JAMA 274:1677-82, 1995.

Suggested Readings

American Medical Association. Good care of the dying patient. *JAMA* 275:474–478, 1994.

Brookshire RH. *An Introduction to Neurogenic Communication Disorders.* St. Louis: Mosby-Year Book, 1992.

Damasio AR. Aphasia. *New England Journal of Medicine* 326:531–539, 1992.

Chapter 11

Communicating with Children About Medicines

Betsy L. Sleath and Patricia J. Bush

Need for Educating Children
and Their Parents About
Medicine

Importance of Using a Patient-
Centered Interaction Style
with Children and Their
Parents

Understanding the Cognitive
Developmental Level of a
Child

General Principles for
Communicating with
Children

Toddlers and Preschool
Children

School-Aged Children

Adolescents

▨ OVERVIEW

Children are important consumers of medicines. Communicating with children is
different from communicating with adults in two distinct ways. First, communication with children typically involves three people: the pharmacist, the child,
and the parent of the child. Second, when educating children about medicines,
one needs to communicate at a level that is appropriate for the cognitive developmental level of the child. This chapter discusses the following areas: (a) the
need for educating children and their parents about medicine, (b) the importance
of using a patient-centered style with children and parents, (c) how to understand
the cognitive developmental level of a child, (d) strategies for communicating
effectively with children at different ages about their medicines, and (e) what children want to know about their medicines at different ages.

Need for Educating Children and Their Parents About Medicine

If you refer to the interpersonal communication model in Chapter 1, you can see that when you communicate about children's medicines, you are potentially sending messages to two receivers—a child and a parent. Ranelli and colleagues (2000) found in a study of Wyoming pharmacists that pharmacists reported considerable contact with children and their families and that most pharmacists (87%) reported filling prescriptions for children daily. However, when Ranelli and colleagues asked the pharmacists whether they communicated directly with children, 33% claimed they did so most of the time, 32% reported doing so some of the time, and 35% reported that they rarely communicated with the child. However, most pharmacists reported that children should become more active participants in the medication process.

When parents come in to purchase prescriptions or over-the-counter medicines for their children, it is important to consider educating the child as well as the parent about the medicine. An advantage to communicating directly with the child is that you are more likely to speak at a level the parent will understand.

There is evidence that children do not receive much education about medicines from physicians or pharmacists. Ranelli and colleagues found that 83% of pharmacists reported that physicians give little information about medicines to children. Menacker et al (1999) interviewed 85 healthy public schoolchildren grades kindergarten through eighth grade and found that most children reported learning about medicines from their mother. The children **reported** that physicians and pharmacists played a limited role in *educating* them about medicines. Most children reported that they *would* ask the doctor or pharmacist a question about medicine but they reported never doing so. The results suggest that pharmacists need to encourage children to ask questions about their medicines. The easiest way to do this is to say to a child "Nearly everyone who gets a medicine has questions about it, including grownups. I bet you have questions, too. Can you tell me a question you have about your medicines?"

There is also evidence that pharmacists need to make sure to educate children about over-the-counter medicines. Bush and Davidson (1982) examined the amount of autonomy that 64 urban children in kindergarten through sixth grades exhibited when it came to medicine taking. They found that nearly 20% of the children reported purchasing over-the-counter medications by themselves. Older children and children in the less economically advantaged neighborhoods were more likely to buy the medicines by themselves. The researchers also found that of the children who reported taking a medicine "yesterday or today," 75% said they took the medicine by themselves, and 40% said they got the medicine by themselves from somewhere in the house. In a follow-up study of 300 urban schoolchildren in grades three through seven, 25% of the children reported purchasing an over-the-counter medicine independently, and 37% reported they had picked up a prescription independently (Iannotti and Bush, 1992).

Pharmacists need to better educate parents about their children's medicines. Ranelli and colleagues (2000) found that 42% of pharmacists reported that physicians give parents little information about medicines. As pharmacists, you need to make sure that parents are informed about their children's medicines to prevent errors from occurring. If you think about the many different strengths of infant and children's acetaminophen and ibuprofen that are available in pharmacies and the many different types of pediatric cough and cold products that are for sale in pharmacies, you can begin to understand how parents can become confused. Pharmacists need to assess what parents know about their child's prescription and over-the-counter medicines by using open-ended questions and then filling in the gaps with education. You can apply the principles you learned in Chapter 8 about building better patient understanding by using them when interacting with both parents and their children about their medicines.

Importance of Using a Patient-Centered Interaction Style with Children and Their Parents

It is important to communicate with both parents and children about medicines. Unfortunately, there has been very little research on pharmacist–parent–child communication (Ranelli et al, 2000). Therefore, to further understand why it is important to educate both parents and children, we need to examine some of the previous work on pediatrician–child–parent communication. Wissow and colleagues (1998) examined physician–parent–child communication about asthma during emergency room visits and found that children took little part in discussions. However, the researchers did find that if physicians used a patient-centered style with children, this was associated with five times more talk with children and higher parent ratings of good care. A patient-centered style is one in which the physician seeks the child's opinions about treatment.

Box 11.1 presents ways to use a patient-centered interaction style. Previous work in both adults and children has shown that patients are more adherent to medicine regimens and have better outcomes if they are taught about their disease and are included in treatment decisions

> **Box 11.1** PATIENT-CENTERED INTERACTION WITH CHILDREN
>   AND PARENTS
>
> • Investigate any concerns or fears both the child and parent
>   might have about the medicine.
> • Ask both the child and parent about priorities for improved
>   quality of life.
> • If the child is on continued therapy, assess how well both the
>   child and parent perceive the medicine is working.
> • Offer to call the pediatrician to suggest possible changes in
>   therapy (if needed based on what you learn from the child and
>   parent).
> • Ask both the child and parent what questions they have about
>   the medicine.
> • Educate both the child and parent about the medicine.

(Adams et al, 2001; Kelly and Scott, 1990; Stewart, 1995; Stewart et al, 2000; Street et al, 1993).

Understanding the Cognitive Developmental Level of a Child

A discussion of the developmental level of children will help you understand how to educate children at different ages and developmental levels about their medicines. Children progress through four stages as they develop cognitive skills. The classification of the four stages is based on the work of Jean Piaget (1932), who examined the development of thinking skills in children. The four stages of cognitive development are (a) the sensory motor stage, (b) the pre-operational stage, (c) the concrete operational stage, and (d) the formal operational stage. It is very important to remember that not all children pass through the stages at the same rate.

The sensory motor stage lasts from birth to roughly 2 years of age. During this stage, all learning is centered around the child, and there is little connection to objects outside the self. Learning about medicines is not really possible in this stage. Learning about medicines does become possible in the later stages.

The pre-operational stage lasts from about age 2 to 7 years. During this stage, children can consider only a single aspect of a situation. Their reasoning is connected to the concrete reality of the here and now. Cause-and-effect relationships are difficult for pre-operational children to understand, so children at this stage will see no connection between their own health and health-related behaviors (e.g., taking a prescribed medicine) (Lau and Klepper, 1988).

The concrete operations stage lasts from about age 7 through 12 years. During this stage, children begin to distinguish between the internal and external worlds. They can use symbols to represent concrete objects and perform mental operations in their head. They can focus on multiple aspects of a situation at one time, and they become problem solvers. However, situations are best presented to them in a concrete or observable manner (O'Brien and Bush, 1993). During this stage, children begin to understand that disease is preventable, and their understanding of health and illness incorporates internal physiological characteristics.

The formal operations stage typically goes from age 13 through adulthood. As children move into adolescence, they become capable of hypothetical and abstract thought. They can reason logically, and their understanding of how one gets sick becomes more realistic. Adolescents begin to develop increased awareness of degrees of illness as well as personal control of one's health.

You need to ask children open-ended questions when they come into the pharmacy. Closed-ended questions provide little information because a child will just answer yes or no. A child's answer to a pharmacist's open-ended questions should reveal their cognitive level (O'Brien and Bush, 1993). After you determine a child's cognitive level, you can adapt how you communicate with them. Box 11.2 presents suggestions of what you could say to children at each stage of cognitive development.

General Principles for Communicating with Children

After a discussion of some basic information about the cognitive development of children, a discussion of different strategies you can use when interacting with children of different ages is helpful. Some children as young as 3 or 4 years and most children by the age 7 or 8 can actively participate in and contribute during visits with health care providers (Behrman and Vaughan, 1983; O'Brien and Bush, 1993). Bush (1996) suggests the following general strategies for communicating with children about medicines:

1. Attempt to communicate at the child's developmental level.
2. Ask open-ended questions rather than questions requiring only a "yes" or "no" response so that you can assess what the child understands.
3. Use simple declarative sentences for all children.
4. Ask the child whether he or she has questions for you.
5. Augment verbal communication with written communication.

Nonverbal communication is very important to children. Children attend to and interpret nonverbal communication before they understand the meanings of words (Behrman and Vaughan, 1983). If you think about it, much of the communication between children and parents is nonverbal (e.g., hugs, sounds, gestures). Therefore, when you interact with children, you need to be aware of your facial expressions, tone of voice, and gestures (Behrman and Vaughan, 1983). Also, try to get down to their level when speaking with them.

Next, we are going to discuss specific communication strategies to use with children of different ages. We will assume that interactions with children typically begin once a child is about 2 years of age and has moved into the pre-operational stage of development. Box 11.3 outlines what children want to know about medicines at different ages.

Box 11.2 COMMUNICATION STRATEGIES FOR DIFFERENT STAGES OF COGNITIVE DEVELOPMENT

Pre-operational (age 2 to 7 years)

Sample educational message: The medicine you'll get will go into your body and make your throat feel better. It will work only if you take it 3 times every day. Your mom will help you know when to take the medicine and when to stop taking the medicine. Be sure to use all the medicine, even if you think you're feeling better.

Concrete operational stage (age 7 to 12 years)

Sample educational message: This medicine will go into your body to help fight off the germs that are causing the infection in your throat. The medicine will work only if you take it 3 times a day until...(date treatment should end). If you don't take it this way, the infection might come back. So keep taking the medicine, even if you think you're feeling better. Work with your mom or dad, so you both know you have taken the medicine at the right times.

Formal operations stage (ages 13 years to adulthood)

Sample educational message: The medicine you're getting will go into your system to help your immune system fight off bacteria that are causing your infection. You have strep throat, which is when a particular form of bacteria causes an irritation in your throat. The medicine used to treat these bacteria is an antibiotic. You have to take it every 8 hours—that is, 3 times a day—for the next 10 days. If you don't do this, there is a chance you will be reinfected. Keep taking your medicine until it is gone, even if you think your throat is better.

From O'Brien R, Bush P. Helping children learn how to use medicines. *Office Nurse* 6: 14–19, 1993.

Box 11.3 WHAT CHILDREN WANT TO KNOW ABOUT
MEDICINES AT DIFFERENT AGES

Children Grades Kindergarten Through First Grade

1. Why some medicines are only for children
2. How they can tell the difference between medicines for children and medicines for adults
3. The therapeutic purposes of medicines (e.g., prevention, cure, symptomatic relief)
4. Dose forms and ways of taking medicines
5. Importance of complying with the treatment regimen
6. The side effects of some medicines
7. That whether a medicine helps is not related to its color, size, or taste

Children Grades Two Through Five

1. What the ingredients (active and inactive) are in medicines
2. How medicines work; where medicines go in the body
3. How doctors know that a medicine works
4. Why there are different medicines for different illnesses
5. Why the same medicine can be for different illnesses
6. Why there are different medicines for a single illness
7. Why you should not take other people's medicines

Children Grades Sixth Through Eighth

1. Difference between prescription and over-the-counter (OTC) medicines
2. Meaning of dependency and addiction
3. How medicines are made
4. Why medicines come in different forms
5. Why one may have to adhere to a special diet and time schedule when taking a medicine
6. Potential for drug interactions with other medicines and foods
7. Lack of a relationship between the efficacy of a medicine and its source or price
8. Difference between brand and generic medicines
9. Difference between medicines, botanicals/herbs, and homeopathics
10. How to select an appropriate over-the-counter medicine
11. For children born outside of the United States or whose parents are recent immigrants: Differences between medicines produced in their country of origin and medicines produced elsewhere

Reprinted from Bush PJ. *Guide to Developing and Evaluating Medicine Education Programs and Materials for Children and Adolescents.* Kent, Ohio: America School Health Association, 1999. Copyright United States Pharmacopeial Convention.

Toddlers and Preschool Children

Although toddlers and preschool children may not be as actively involved in learning about medicines as older children, it is important to include them in discussions about their medicines. A good way to begin an encounter with toddlers and preschool children is to start with a simple friendly greeting and then do an enthusiastic but brief examination of one of the child's toys (Coulehan and Block, 1992). In Ranelli's study (2000), a pharmacist reported special tactics for dealing with children. "It's good to have an icebreaker for kids. I always have a stash of bouncy balls and do a 'magic trick.' Once one has gained their attention and confidence, giving instructions becomes much easier." At this age, it is important to begin educating children as to what the medicine is for and why it is important to take it in simple terms.

Another pharmacist in Ranelli's study commented on his son's diagnosis with asthma at age 3, "Even then he understood why the medicine was important and when he needed a puff. He was in charge of his inhalers from second grade on because he was too shy to go to the school nurse." At this age, you want the child to feel that taking medicines is important. However, you also want to emphasize that the child should not take medicines without permission from mom or dad. You could do something as simple as letting the child put a label on the prescription. This way the child will know it is his or her own medicine.

School-Aged Children

When children reach the age of 5 or 6 years, they can be more actively involved when you educate them and their parents about their medicines. A good way to begin an interaction may be to ask the child about his or her favorite television show or hobby (Coulehan and Block, 1992). There can be a huge developmental range among elementary school children and great differences in their experiences with medicines, which is why you need to ask children open-ended questions to assess their cognitive level and knowledge. Through some simple questions such as "Why do you need to take this medicine?" or "How does the medicine work?" you can assess whether the child is starting to understand cause-and-effect relationships and that internal physiological mechanisms contribute toward illness. If we consider Piaget's work, this typically happens around age 7, but it can happen when a child is younger or older.

Once a child begins to understand cause-and-effect relationships, you can give the child more details about how a medicine works in the body. You can also start to give the child more autonomy in medicine taking by saying "work with your mom or dad in taking the medicine" instead of "do not take the medicine unless your mom or dad is present." At this age, you also need to talk with the parent to ascertain how independent the child is becoming in medicine taking.

Children with chronic conditions such as diabetes, epilepsy, or asthma may have a very good understanding of their disease and medicines. Box 11.3 presents what schoolchildren indicated they want to know about their medicines at different ages (Bush, 1999).

Adolescents

When children reach adolescence, you may want to spend part of the time communicating with the adolescent without the parents present. Pediatricians often ask parents to leave the room so they can communicate privately with adolescent children. Pharmacists can use the same technique. This allows you to build trust with the patient. Trust becomes especially important with adolescents. An adolescent may feel comfortable talking with you about birth control and sexually transmitted diseases if you sometimes talk with them independently of their parents. Adolescents need to know you will not tell their parents what they say or what they buy. In general, you can typically give teenagers educational messages that would be equivalent to what you would give an adult.

SUMMARY

It is important to make sure that both parents and children are appropriately educated about their medicines. Pharmacists need to make sure to use a "patient-centered" interaction style when interacting with parents and children. Also, pharmacists need to remember to assess the cognitive developmental level of children through the use of open-ended questions. At the national level, the *United States Pharmacopoeia* has a position statement called "Ten Guiding Principles for Teaching Children and Adolescents about Medicines," which supports the right of children and adolescents to receive developmentally appropriate information and direct communications about medicines (Bush et al, 1999). Four of these ten guiding principles relate to pharmacist–parent–child communication. These four principles are an excellent summary of what you have learned in this chapter:

1. Children want to know. Health care providers and health educators should communicate directly with children about medicines.

2. Children's interest should be encouraged, and they should be taught how to ask questions of health care providers, parents, and other caregivers about medicines and other therapies.

3. Children, their parents, and their health care providers should negotiate the gradual transfer of responsibility for medicine use in ways that respect parental responsibilities and the health status and capabilities of the child.

4. Children's medicine education should take into account what children want to know about medicines, as well as what health care professionals think children should know.

REVIEW QUESTIONS

1. Describe the "patient-centered" interaction style involved with medication therapy for children.

2. What are the four stages of cognitive development proposed by Piaget?

3. What educational strategies would you use in each of Piaget's development phases?

4. Based on past research, what type of information should be the focus when educating a 7-year-old child about his or her medications?

REVIEW EXERCISE

After reading through the sample educational messages contained in Box 11.2, write down how the content of the message changed at each stage and how this reflects the cognitive level of the child. Next, pretend that you need to verbally educate a child at each stage of cognitive development about their diabetes medicines. Write down what you would say to a child at each different level of development.

References

Adams RJ, Smith BJ, Ruffin R. Impact of the physician's participatory style in asthma outcomes and patient satisfaction. *Annals of Allergy, Asthma & Immunology* 86:263–271, 2001.

Behrman RE, Vaughan VC III. *Textbook of Pediatrics*. Philadelphia: WB Saunders, 1983.

Bush PJ. Children and medicines. In Smith MC, Wertheimer AI, eds. *Social and Behavioral Aspects of Pharmaceutical Care*. Binghamton, NY: Pharmaceutical Products Press, 1996:449–471.

Bush PJ. *Guide to Developing and Evaluating Medicine Education Programs and Materials for Children and Adolescents*. Kent, Ohio: America School Health Association, 1999.

Bush PJ, Davidson FR. Medicines and "drugs": what do children think? *Health Education Quarterly* 9:113–128, 1982.

Bush PJ, Ozias JM, Walson PD, Ward RM. Ten guiding principles for teaching children and adolescents about medicines. *Clinical Therapeutics* 21:1280–1284, 1999.

Coulehan JL, Block MR. *The Medical Interview: A Primer for Students of the Art.* Philadelphia: FA Davis, 1992.

Kelly GR, Scott JE. Medication compliance and health education among outpatients with chronic mental disorders. *Medical Care* 28:1181–1197, 1990.

Lau RR, Klepper S. The development of illness orientations in children aged 6 through 12. *Journal of Health and Social Behavior* 29:149–168, 1988.

Menacker F, Aramburuzabala P, Minian N, Bush P, Bibace R. Children and medicines: what they want to know and how they want to learn. *Journal of Social and Administrative Pharmacy.* 16:38-52, 1999.

O'Brien R, Bush P. Helping children learn how to use medicines. *Office Nurse* 6:14–19, 1993.

Piaget J. *The Moral Judgement of the Child.* New York: Harcourt, Brace, and World, Inc, 1932.

Ranelli P, Bartsch K, London K. Pharmacists' perceptions of children and families as medicine consumers. *Psychology and Health* 15:829–840, 2000.

Stewart M. Effective physician-patient communication and health outcomes: a review. *Canadian Medical Association Journal* 152:1423–1433, 1995.

Stewart M, Meredith L, Brown JB, Galajda J. The influence of older patient-physician communication on health and health-related outcomes. *Clinics in Geriatric Medicine* 16:25–36, 2000.

Street R, Piziak V, Carpentier W, et al. Provider-patient communication and metabolic control. *Diabetes Care* 16:714–721, 1993.

Wissow L, Roter D, Bauman LJ, et al. Patient-provider communication during the emergency department care of children with asthma. *Medical Care* 36:1439–1450, 1998.

Chapter 12

Ethical Issues in Patient Counseling

Ethical Patient Care

Ethical Principles

Patient–Provider Relationships

Resolving Ethical Dilemmas

Analyzing Patient Cases

▨ OVERVIEW

In the context of patient counseling, pharmacists have ethical obligations to patients and to society. To know how to resolve ethical issues and to make ethical decisions, pharmacists must understand general ethical principles and their applications to patient care situations. This chapter outlines key principles relevant to pharmacist–patient relationships and presents a decision-making process to assist pharmacists in resolving ethical conflicts.

Ethical Patient Care

The following cases illustrate several principles of ethical behavior discussed in this chapter. As you read the following three cases, make notes about what you would do in each situation. The cases are reviewed later in the chapter.

CASE 1: Ms. Edwards is starting on a new medication for schizophrenia. The drug has a number of side effects, some of which can be serious. She asks you several questions about the purpose of the medication and possible side effects. When you ask her what her physician told her about the medication, she reports that he said "I've got a lot of patients on this drug and they're doing fine." It is obvious to you that she is unclear about the purpose of the medication or any possible problems.

You are concerned that Ms. Edwards may refuse to take the drug if told about possible side effects. What would you say to Ms. Edwards?

CASE 2: To fulfill regulations requiring pharmacists to offer counseling to patients, the manager of the pharmacy that you just started working in has trained pharmacy clerks to say to patients in a neutral tone of voice "It may be a while before you can talk with a pharmacist about your medications. Do you really want to talk with the pharmacist?" When you learn of this approach, you argue with your manager that this approach is inadequate and that you want to talk with patients personally. You insist that this is the only way you can verify that they understand how to use their medications and be aware of potential problems. The manager states that counseling is not required under current regulations when patients decline the offer to counsel. Furthermore, he says, the store is too busy to go beyond these minimum requirements and is financially having trouble surviving the intense competition in the area as it is. He also states that he encourages pharmacists to counsel patients in depth if they have time and if no other patients are waiting for their prescriptions. What are the ethical principles involved with this situation? How would you handle this dilemma?

CASE 3: James Bently, a 17-year-old patient of your pharmacy, was diagnosed with epilepsy and was prescribed phenytoin about 6 months ago. In conversations with him, you have discovered that he considers epilepsy embarrassing and has indicated that he does not believe his physician is correct in the diagnosis. James expressed his belief that he does not really need the drug. Your refill records indicate a pattern of nonadherence to the medication. In the past, you have tried to educate him about phenytoin and the importance of consistent use in controlling seizures. However, he still does not take the drug as prescribed. James also continues to drive his car and you are aware that he was recently charged in a non-injury automobile accident. His father, who occasionally picks up the medication for James, has never indicated awareness of his son's denial of epilepsy or noncompliance with treatment. Should you disclose the fact that James is not taking his medication to his father, to the police, or to his physician?

Each of these patient cases presents decisions that must be made on the basis of legal and ethical principles. Your ability to choose a proper course of action in these situations depends on your understanding of these principles. The legal aspects of these cases are covered under state and federal law. However, many elements are not specifically addressed in laws and regulations but do involve underlying ethical principles of patient–health professional interaction. Principles related to ethical decision making in patient care include beneficence, autonomy, and honesty (Beauchamp and Childers, 1989; Van deVeer and Regan, 1987; Veatch, 1989). This is by no means a complete list, but the principles seem to be most relevant to the communication responsibilities of phar-

Box 12.1 ETHICAL PRINCIPLES

- Beneficence
- Autonomy
- Honesty

- Informed consent
- Confidentiality
- Fidelity

macists. Other issues that are derived from these principles and are particularly important in patient counseling are informed consent, confidentiality, and fidelity.

Ethical Principles

Box 12.1 summarizes key ethical principles of communication for health professionals.

Beneficence

Beneficence is the principle that health professionals should act in the best interest of the patient. The principle of beneficence is found in the Hippocratic oath, which states that physicians will apply measures "for the benefit of the sick according to my ability and judgment." Beneficence is also addressed in the APhA Code of Ethics (1994), "A pharmacist places concern for the well-being of the patient at the center of professional practice."

Examinations of medical ethics have highlighted the dangers of beneficence—dangers that threaten individual rights and personal liberties. In the past, medicine has used the beneficence principle as justification for a "paternalistic" relationship with patients. Physicians made decisions by themselves (without necessarily informing patients and without patient consent) as to what was in the patient's best interest. They made certain decisions based on their perceptions as to what was needed and did not include patients in this decision making. In recent years, standards for patient care emphasize patient autonomy and support the right of patients to decide for themselves whether treatment is or is not in the patient's own best interest.

Autonomy

The principle of autonomy establishes patient rights to self-determination—to choose what will be done to them. This right is considered paramount even if health professionals judge patient decisions as being damaging to their health. It is helpful to evaluate ethical dilemmas in light of the patient autonomy–paternalistic continuum. Some actions are more authoritarian than others and thus would be placed toward the "paternalistic" end of this continuum. Actions that encourage patient involvement in decision making would be placed toward the "patient autonomy" end of this continuum. It is also important to assess an individual's perceptions of certain actions. For example, patients may view a particular action as being more paternalistic than do health care providers. These differences in perceptions may lead to strained patient–provider relationships.

Honesty

The honesty principle states that patients have the right to the truth about their medical condition, the course of their disease, the treatments recommended, and alternative treatments available. The APhA Code of Ethics (1994) states that a pharmacist "has a duty to tell the truth and to act with conviction of conscience." A certain level of trust must develop between patients and pharmacists to strengthen these relationships. This trust is built on the principle of honesty.

Informed Consent

Both honesty and autonomy serve as foundations to the right of the patient to give informed consent to treatment. The informed consent principle states that patients have the right to full disclosure of all relevant aspects of care and must give explicit consent to treatment before treatment is initiated (Beauchamp, 1989; Brock, 1987). Informed consent has occurred and treatment can be implemented in the following situations:

1. If all relevant information is provided
2. If patients understand the information
3. If consent is freely given and is without coercion
4. If patients are capable of understanding the salient information
5. If patients give consent to a particular treatment

Unfortunately, many times in actual practice, health care professionals focus more on "disclosure" than on patient understanding of information. The term "informed consent" requires an acceptable level of patient understanding as a more essential component than disclosure per se. Beauchamp (1989) summarizes this position: "the central problems about informed consent are issues of communication rather than the abstract and disembodied issues about proper legal standards of disclosure." He also states: "the key to effective communication is to invite participation by patients or subjects in an exchange of information and disclosure. Asking questions, eliciting the concerns and interests of patients, and establishing a climate that encourages patients to ask questions may be more important than the full corpus of disclosed information." It is insufficient, given the above definition of informed consent, for health care providers to be "available" to consult or respond to questions.

A meaningful dialogue or consent process is unlikely to be initiated by patients themselves for a variety of reasons. This is true in part because of patient reticence to question providers. In addition, patients often cannot *know* when there is important information about treatment that they have not yet acquired. The burden is on providers to *make sure* that patients understand all they need to know both to make a reasoned decision about therapy and to implement therapeutic plans appropriately.

Drug therapy is the most common type of treatment in health care. However, informed consent issues surrounding medication use are largely ignored compared with issues involving other types of treatment, such as surgery. In addition, patients have much more control over management of their medication therapy. Earlier assumptions by society that risks associated with drug therapy are minimal have been challenged by recent research (IOM, 2001). The estimated number of deaths and adverse health events caused by inappropriate therapy is staggering. In the future, pharmacists will be expected to assume their share of responsibility in ensuring that informed consent has occurred before drug treatment is initiated.

What are the roles of pharmacists in informed consent? Many pharmacists assume that when patients bring in prescriptions, (a) their physicians have provided all relevant information, (b) patients understand the information, and (c) they have consented to treatment. In fact, research has shown that many patients lack information on crucial aspects of drug treatment (Semla et al, 1991). In addition, physicians frequently do not explicitly discuss key aspects of drug therapy and often fail to obtain meaningful consent from patients.

In many situations, it is obvious that informed consent has really *not* occurred. Patients may not fully understand important aspects of treatment, may have unanswered questions, or may not be aware of significant side effects. In addition, patients may indicate reluctance to begin taking medications but feel that they have no choice but to follow their physicians' directions. Many may feel coerced into their decision based on the hierarchical relationship between patient and provider, where power is largely vested in the health professionals on whom patients feel dependent. It is difficult to determine whether consent to treatment has been freely given. When patients express reservations about initiating drug treatment, pharmacists may need to consult not only with patients but also with prescribing physicians to inform them of the lack of freely given consent to treatment.

Confidentiality

The principle of confidentiality serves to assure patients that information about their medical conditions and treatments will not be given to individuals without their permission. Brody (1989) makes the case that confidentiality is "central to preserving the human dignity of patients." He explains that a large part of patients' sense of control over their lives is wrapped up in their ability to choose to whom they wish to reveal their most personal selves and what information they wish to confide. Self-disclosure is the essence of intimacy in relationships and patients desire control over this personal act.

The relationship between patient and health provider circumvents the normal progression of intimate relationships. Patients are expected to divulge the most personal details to health care providers, who may be virtual strangers. To maintain the reciprocal trust that is essential in these relationships, professionals must be able to trust the truthfulness of patient reports, and patients must be able to trust that this information will not be shared with others not involved in their medical care.

Fidelity

Fidelity is the right of patients to have health professionals provide services that promote patients' interests rather than their own. Pharmacists who encourage the use of vitamins that patients do not need may be promoting their financial well-being at the expense of the patients. Pharmacists who refuse to confront physicians about inappropriate prescribing because they want to ensure that physicians will continue to direct patients to their pharmacies are displaying a misplaced sense of their professional responsibility. Pharmacists who are more attentive to the desires of the parties signing their paychecks than to the health care needs of their patients are in a conflict-of-interest situation. Ethically, the responsibilities of pharmacists should be directed toward the welfare of patients.

Patient–Provider Relationships

The focus on rights of patients and obligations of providers can make the relationships between them seem mechanistic and legalistic. It would be easy to create a list of dos and don'ts for each party to follow. However, the situations encountered in the patient–provider relationship are often complicated. Thus, the principles discussed above must be considered when working with patients. In addition, the ability to effectively work through sensitive issues depends on trusting, caring relationships between patients and providers. Each patient is a unique individual and, in an illness situation, is particularly vulnerable. Thus, patients have the right to be treated with compassion. Patients need humane, sensitive care from providers, care that will assist them in making the best decisions they are able to make (Fried, 1974). This is the essence of the "helping" role of the health care professional.

Brody (1992) makes the case that the vulnerability of the patient and the status accorded physicians and other health professionals set up a power difference fraught with danger for the patient. He states, "if one shares the power with the person in greatest danger of being victimized, the potential for self-correction of error seems greatest." Once again, the need for mutual participation and an active patient role in health care decision making becomes essential. Empowering patients to be active participants in treatment decisions, with decisions being made in the context of a respectful, trusting relationship, is a large part of our professional responsibility to patients.

Resolving Ethical Dilemmas

The steps involved in reaching ethical decisions are essentially identical with those used in resolving other professional or general moral dilemmas (Box 12.2). To become more familiar with this ethical decision process, you are encouraged to read case studies in the pharmacy literature (Veatch and Haddad, 1999) or attend ethics courses in colleges of pharmacy or through continuing education programs. These experiences may assist you in practicing this important decision-making process so that you become more efficient in making real life decisions.

Analyzing Patient Cases

Three patient cases began this chapter that present ethical dilemmas to pharmacists. Here, each case is analyzed in the following text according to the ethical principles involved.

Case 1

It is obvious that Ms. Edwards does not understand the purpose of drug treatment nor the medication's possible side effects. Thus, it could be argued that she has not actually given informed consent to treatment. Arguments against providing information may revolve around fears that Ms. Edwards may not take the medication she needs to treat her medical condition if she is aware of the side effects. The principle

---

Box 12.2 STEPS IN ETHICAL DECISION MAKING

Experience has shown that the following steps may be helpful in reaching a decision:

1. Recognize and state the ethical dilemma(s) involved in a situation or case.
2. Collect all relevant facts including both medical as well as social/psychological aspects of the case. These facts may clarify whether the problem really does involve ethical issues or not.
3. If the problem involves ethical issues, generate all possible alternatives to resolving the ethical dilemma.
4. Evaluate alternatives in terms of principles that apply as well as possible consequences of the different choices. One exercise that is useful is to provide principle-based justification for all alternatives, arguing on either side of an ethical dilemma.
5. Choose the best alternative (or combine alternatives), and justify your choice in terms of the prioritization of ethical principles involved. Often one principle must be suspended in favor of a more compelling principle in resolving a dilemma.
6. Recommend a specific course of action.

---

invoked in such a case is beneficence—doing something that you decide is in her best interest. Other arguments against informing Ms. Edwards may focus on the physician, on beliefs that it is the physician's responsibility to inform patients or the physician's right to choose not to provide her with certain information about her treatment. Other arguments may focus on your fears about antagonizing physicians by acting contrary to their wishes and jeopardizing physician referrals to the pharmacy.

The principle of autonomy and the right of the patient to determine what will be done to her body argue in favor of your providing information about the medication, including its purpose and side effects. You may need to call Ms. Edwards' physician to gather further information pertinent to her treatment or to consult with the physician on how informed consent should take place. Nevertheless, Ms. Edwards has the right to this information and must be informed before she begins taking the medication.

This case highlights the potential conflict of interest facing you in which self-interest or allegiances to others (e.g., physicians) are allowed to override the interests of your patients. The right of the patient to fidelity in the patient–pharmacist relationship is threatened by such a position. You may put yourself in a compromised position to take the physicians' position over the patient's needs. Although the principles of beneficence and autonomy may be in conflict in this case, the right of self-determination by the patient is so fundamental as to be paramount. Ms. Edwards has the right to information about her medication, regardless of whether that information would affect her decision to initiate treatment.

Case 2

The second example, in which your manager wants his employees to curtail patient counseling, clearly identifies a potential conflict of interest. Your self-interest (pleasing your boss, keeping harmony in the workplace) is pitted against the patient's need for information about prescribed medications. One of the defining characteristics of health professionals is to hold the needs of patients above all else. Whenever the amount of consultation is based on considerations *other* than patient need (e.g., I was too busy, there were too many other patients waiting), the decision is contrary to several of the ethical principles discussed above. Thus, time should be allocated to counseling patients who need the personal interaction with you. Patients will appreciate your efforts. How you allocate your time in practice reveals a lot about your underlying ethical principles.

Case 3

Case 3 involves a decision on whether to reveal confidential information (that James is not taking his antiseizure medication regimen) to other parties. The injunction against release of information without patient consent is strongly held and is based in part on the patient's right of self-determination. It is up to James to decide what information is transmitted to other parties about his medical treatment. The argument for breaking confidentiality in this situation rests on the principle of beneficence (acting in the best interests of James by preventing him from injuring himself in an automobile accident). In fact, you may be justified in breaking confidentiality by invoking a duty to protect innocent people (e.g., those potentially injured in future automobile accidents). However, a decision to inform parents and the police would appear to break confidentiality between James and you. Thus, you may not want to approach these individuals.

One approach may be to press James to allow you to discuss the situation with his parents so that they can participate in this complex process. This motivation would be based on your desire (beneficence) to help James with his treatment. Informing James' physician would generally not be considered a breach of confidentiality, since the physician initiated treatment and since medical information can legitimately be shared with other health professionals involved in a patient's care. Possibly James' physician and you could discuss how to approach James and his parents about this important issue.

Additional Case

For more practice in analyzing ethical situations, here is an additional case to review.

> You are working as a relief pharmacist in a community pharmacy. You notice that Megan, the 17-year-old daughter of a very close family friend, is receiving prescriptions for oral contraceptives and for the treatment of a sexually transmitted disease (STD). Apparently, Megan has been hanging out with a group of students whom her parents disapprove of and have forbidden her to see. You are very concerned about Megan and wonder whether her use of oral contraceptives may lead her to forego the use of condoms that could offer protection from STDs. When Megan enters the pharmacy to pick up her prescriptions, she becomes upset at seeing you and hurries out, refusing to talk to you. You know that if you were in her parents' shoes, you would want to know about the prescriptions. You are convinced that Megan is in trouble and needs the help of her family.

Consider the following questions: What is the ethical dilemma? What additional facts may be needed to help you reach a decision in this case? What alternatives might you consider in resolving this dilemma? What ethical principles are involved in the decision? What alternative would you choose and why? How would you proceed in carrying out your decision?

In listing the ethical principles involved with this case, you probably identified patient confidentiality and beneficence as two of the most important principles. The first principle implies that, as a pharmacist, you must protect the confidential nature of the patient–provider relationship and therefore must not discuss this issue with Megan's parents. On the other hand, this may conflict with your need to do something to act in Megan's best interest (beneficence). You may feel compelled to tell her parents (since she is a minor) and get them involved in dealing with Megan's medical, psychological, and social issues.

In evaluating each approach, the confidentiality issues appear to be clearer than the beneficence issues. Confidentiality simply states that you should not tell Megan's parents without her consent. You may resolve the confidentiality issue by urging Megan to grant you permission to speak with her parents based on your appeal that in the long run it will be the best for all parties concerned. The beneficence

REVIEW CASE 12.1

A patient confides in you that his cardiologist "twisted his arm" to enroll in a clinical trial of a new medication for congestive heart failure that the physician is testing for the drug company. The patient tells you that he did not really want to be a "guinea pig" but said that he did not want to make his cardiologist mad at him either, since "my life is in his hands."

What are the ethical principles involved in this case?

What would you say to this patient?

What would your role be in this situation?

issues are more complex, since you need to identify the real underlying issues. You must ask yourself, "Am I really looking out for Megan's interest or am I responding to my own parental instincts." In addition, you may be responding out of fear of what would happen if Megan's parents eventually found out that you knew about her situation. Fear of losing friends and their business should not be the primary motivators in this situation. Pharmacists may certainly break confidentiality when a patient's life is in danger, such as when concerns about suicide exist. However, resolving a confidentiality issue when the threat to a patient's health is more psychological than physical is more difficult.

SUMMARY

Pharmacists must understand the principles that serve as foundations for ethical decisions in health care. The obligation to respect patient autonomy, to protect confidentiality of patient information, to serve patient welfare, and to treat patients with respect and compassion are fundamental duties for any health care professional. Use of a systematic decision-making process when ethical dilemmas arise and principles seem to compete can assist you in reaching decisions that are ethically valid.

REVIEW QUESTIONS

1. Describe "beneficence" and compare it with "fidelity."
2. State some of the limitations of "informed consent."
3. Describe a rationale for pharmacists to use in resolving ethical dilemmas.

References

APhA Code of Ethics. American Pharmaceutical Association, adopted by the membership on October 27, 1994.

Beauchamp T. Informed consent. In Veatch RM, ed. *Medical Ethics*. Boston: Jones and Bartlett, 1989.

Beauchamp TL, Childers JF. *Principles of Biomedical Ethics*. New York: Oxford University Press, 1989.

Brock DW. Informed consent. In Van deVeer D, Regan T, eds. *Health Care Ethics*. Philadelphia: Temple University Press, 1987.

Brody H. *The Healer's Power*. New Haven, CT: Yale University Press, 1992.

Brody H. The physician/patient relationship. In Veatch RM, ed. *Medical Ethics*. Boston: Jones and Bartlett, 1989.

Fried C. *Medical Experimentation: Personal Integrity and Social Policy*. New York: American Elsevier, 1974.

Institute of Medicine. *Crossing the Quality Chasm: A New Health System for the 21st Century,* Washington, DC, 2001.

Semla TP, Lemke JH, Helling DK, et al. Perceived purpose of prescription drugs: the Iowa 65+ rural health study. *DICP: Annals of Pharmacotherapy* 25: 410–413, 1991.

Van deVeer D, Regan T, eds. *Health Care Ethics*. Philadelphia: Temple University Press, 1987.

Veatch R. Informed consent: The emerging principles. In Wertheimer AL, Smith MC, eds. *Pharmacy Practice: Social and Behavioral Aspects*, 3rd ed. Baltimore: Williams & Wilkins, 1989: 338.

Veatch R, Haddad A. *Case Studies in Pharmacy Ethics*. New York: Oxford Press, 1999.

Suggested Readings

Brenner J, Beardsley RS. White paper on pharmacy student professionalism. *Journal of the American Pharmaceutical Association* 40 (Jan-Feb):96–102, 2000.

Hepler CD, Strand LM. Opportunities and responsibilities in pharmaceutical care. *American Journal of Hospital Pharmacy* 47: 533–543, 1990.

Self DJ, Baldwin CJ, Wolinsky, FD. Evaluation of teaching medical ethics by an assessment of moral reasoning. *Medical Education* 26: 178–184, 1992.

Self DJ, Wolinsky FD, Baldwin DC. The effect of teaching medical ethics on medical students' moral reasoning. *Academic Medicine* 64: 755–759, 1989.

Wu WC, Pearlman RA. Consent in medical decision-making: the role of communication. *Journal of General Internal Medicine* 3: 9–14, 1988.

Appendix

Application and Critical Analysis

This appendix presents several cases that illustrate certain skills and techniques described in previous chapters. These cases provide an opportunity to critically analyze communication skill development as well as an opportunity to analyze how pharmacists respond to patients. They are examples of how communication may be enhanced by using the various communication skills and techniques discussed in this book. The cases simulate communication problems in actual pharmacy practice. In some, specific communication skills and strategies are described in detail, whereas in others, you are asked to hypothesize what should be done.

Most of these examples involve professional problem solving that may be difficult for people without much pharmacy experience. You may have difficulty responding to some of these cases based on your view of your role in these situations. Many pharmacists may not be involved in some of these situations, but many will. The goal is to analyze each situation, plan a particular strategy, and anticipate a favorable outcome.

Case Study 1

The first case study involves pharmacist Jill Thompson and 4-year-old patient Jim Conrad, who has had several seizures and has recently undergone neurological testing. Mrs. Conrad, Jim's mother, picks up a new prescription for Dilantin Infatabs (phenytoin) for Jim.

> **JILL:** Mrs. Conrad, the prescription for Jim is ready. Before you go, I'd like to spend about 5 minutes discussing this medicine with you. I want to make sure that Jim doesn't run into any problems when he starts taking the medication.
>
> **MRS. CONRAD:** Fine. I have time now.
>
> **JILL:** Let's sit over here where we will have some privacy.
>
> **MRS. CONRAD:** All right.
>
> **JILL:** Mrs. Conrad, your doctor has prescribed Dilantin to treat Jim's epilepsy.

Mrs. Conrad: How did you know he has epilepsy?

Jill: Well. . . that is the most typical diagnosis for the use of this drug.

Mrs. Conrad: I see.

Jill: Jim is supposed to take the Dilantin three times a day. You should space the doses as evenly as possible over a 24-hour period. This will mean that you will be giving the Dilantin every 8 hours.

Mrs. Conrad: I know all that. My doctor went over these instructions quite thoroughly.

Jill: Did he discuss the side effects Jim might have when he begins taking the medicine?

Mrs. Conrad: Yes. He did that quite thoroughly as well.

Jill: Very good. One other thing I am concerned about is establishing a time for taking the medicines that fits into your daily routine. Otherwise, it is very difficult to remember to take the medicine. Let's start with the morning—what time does Jim get up?

Mrs. Conrad: Usually around 6.

Jill: What time does he go to bed?

Mrs. Conrad: About 9.

Jill: If you gave doses at 6 in the morning, at 1:30 in the afternoon and at 9 at night, that would be close enough to every 8 hours. Is there anything you do at 1:30 every day that would help you remember to give Jim his medicine—eat lunch, put him down for a nap, that sort of thing.

Mrs. Conrad: No. We eat lunch at 11:30 and Jim rarely takes a nap anymore.

Jill: You're wearing a digital watch. . .does it have an alarm you can set?

Mrs. Conrad: Yes, it does.

Jill: I recommend setting it to go off when Jim's afternoon dose of medication is due. Otherwise, setting an alarm at your house or posting a note you will be sure to see at 1:30 will help you remember to give Jim that dose. Otherwise, it is very hard to remember to take a medication when you first start using it.

Mrs. Conrad: The watch alarm is a good suggestion. I'm not good at remembering to give him medicine.

Jill: I am giving you a leaflet that tells more about the medicine, including what to do if you forget to give a dose. Please read it carefully and call me if you have any questions or concerns.

MRS. CONRAD: Thank you.

JILL: Are there any questions you have now or issues you would like to discuss?

MRS. CONRAD: I sure hope this medication works. The seizures were awful to see.

JILL: That must have been very frightening for you.

MRS. CONRAD: It was. I was so scared and felt so helpless.

JILL: It has to be hard to learn to cope with such a disease.

MRS. CONRAD: At least now I know what the problem is and how to handle a seizure when it happens.

JILL: This medication helps a lot of people with epilepsy lead normal lives. We'll work with you to get Jim's dosing plan to be just right for him. And please call me if you have any concerns about his treatment once you get home and start giving Jim the medication.

MRS. CONRAD: Thank you.

Take a minute to analyze the above dialogue in terms of the skills and barriers to effective communication discussed earlier in the text. Examine each of Jill's responses and analyze its effect on the communication process. Which of Jill's responses were ineffective and why? How did the patient respond to Jill in these instances? What specifically should Jill have done to improve the communication? What were the positive aspects of Jill's communication? What assertiveness, empathy, interviewing, assessment, and patient education issues are evident in this exchange? How well did Jill meet her ethical responsibilities to the patient? What assumptions did she seem to make that may not have been true?

Let's examine some specific responses by Jill. When she begins the conversation with Mrs. Conrad, Jill calls her by name, tells her that she wishes to discuss the new prescription and why, tells her how long the consultation will take and gets her consent to proceed. Jill is assertive in initiating communication and shows respect for Mrs. Conrad by explaining the purpose of the consultation and getting her cooperation. She also makes sure they have the privacy necessary to facilitate effective communication. These are all positive responses on the part of Jill.

Problems first appear when Jill starts providing information about the new medication. Her assumption that the physician has diagnosed epilepsy seems presumptuous to the patient's mother and she reacts negatively. This problem could have been avoided if Jill had let the mother explain what the physician had told her about the diagnosis and about the new drug treatment. This would have prevented Jill from repeating information about the dosing schedule Mrs. Conrad already knew, which led to impatience on her part. It also would have led to a more thorough assessment of how well informed the mother was about side effects and precautions to follow after Jim begins taking the medication. The closed question, "Did [your physician] discuss the side effects Jim might have," led to a "yes" response, which is an inadequate way of assessing understanding. Asking open-ended questions would have been more efficient. In addition, without verifying that such understanding exists, Jill cannot ensure that informed consent to treatment has taken place.

Jill attempts to tailor the regimen schedule to Jim's daily routine and to suggest cues or reminders to help the mother remember doses. Such an effort will go a long way toward assisting Mrs. Conrad in carrying out the regimen demands. Success in adhering to treatment demands early on leads to increased feelings of self-efficacy or confidence in the ability to follow treatment recommendations on the part of patients or patients' caregivers.

Finally, Jill showed a great deal of understanding for the difficulties Jim's epilepsy presented for the mother. She asked an open-ended question on whether Mrs. Conrad had issues she wished to discuss and was empathic toward her when she expressed her fears and feelings of helplessness. Jill made it clear that she wants to work with Mrs. Conrad in establishing effective treatment for her son and that she is available to her to discuss concerns Mrs. Conrad might have in the future.

Case Study 2

With the limited time available for pharmacist–patient interaction, it is important to decide exactly what to cover during this time period. The following case outlines possible approaches.

You are a new pharmacist practicing in a community pharmacy setting. A patient, Jane Kramer, comes into the pharmacy to get a new prescription filled for Glucotrol XL (glipizide). In checking her patient profile, you learn that she is a longtime patron of the pharmacy, is 55 years old, is 5´4´´ tall and weighs 185 lbs. She has a refill history for Lipitor that indicates a pattern of late refills—in fact, the last refill should have run out two weeks ago. She got a new prescription for Clinoril filled three weeks ago and one for Biaxin two weeks ago. The Lipitor, Clinoril and Glucotrol XL are prescribed by Dr. Sharp and the Biaxin by Dr. Long.

What additional information should be obtained from Jane? What would you want to know about her medical conditions and her medication therapy? What barriers do you think might keep you from getting a complete picture of her medication therapy?

The six points below are offered as potential areas of inquiry in future interactions. Specific examples related to Jane Kramer's case provide additional insight.

1. *Information should be obtained on all prescription and significant nonprescription medications the patient is currently taking in order to ensure that profiles are complete.* If you assume that your computer profile about Ms. Kramer provides a complete picture of current prescription medication use, you may be misled. For example, Jane may be using a Prozac prescription filled in the pharmacy located next door to the psychiatrist. In addition, she may be taking large amounts of aspirin for headaches which may increase the toxicity of Clinoril.

2. *Information should be obtained on the chronic use of medications.* If you automatically assume that the late refills on Lipitor means that she is unwilling to take her medications as prescribed, you would have been mistaken. You find out later that her husband recently lost his job; money is extremely tight; and her physician, knowing this, gave her samples of Lipitor to use as supplements to her prescriptions. The key is to ask open-ended questions to explore this important area. How does Jane actually take these medications? What problems does she perceive with their use? How effective have they seemed to be in terms of results of physician monitoring of lipid levels?

3. *Similarly, you should assess understanding about acute care medications as well.* For example, Jane went to a walk-in clinic approximately two weeks ago and was diagnosed with an upper respiratory infection. She was given a prescription for Biaxin that she was supposed to take twice a day for 10 days. After about 4 or 5 days, she started to feel better and finally quit taking the medication altogether. Although she still had a cough at night, she did not mention this to her primary care physician since she was embarrassed to admit that she had seen a different physician.

4. *During your work up, the possible presence of other medical problems that are not being treated or that her physician is unaware of should be assessed.* In this case, her primary physician is unaware of her lingering cough.

5. *Special emphasis should be placed on any new medication being prescribed for the first time.* In this case, Jane has recently been prescribed Glucotrol XL. You find that she has been trying to control her diabetes with diet and exercise as her physician recommended, but with little success. Now that she is receiving a medication, she is confused about whether she must continue to fol-

low the diet and exercise plan. She appears to be well informed about the treatment, but has misconceptions about the disease and is not optimistic about her ability to control its progression.

6. *Concerns or questions the patient might have about her diseases and/or treatments should be assessed.* In talking with Jane you find that she is extremely upset about her diagnosis of diabetes and discouraged because she has been unable to control it through diet and exercise. Her father had juvenile-onset diabetes and died when she was 10 of renal failure caused by uncontrolled diabetes. Although the physician did tell her that she had a different type of diabetes, her anxiety and an incomplete explanation on the part of the physician caused her to fail to understand the difference between type 1 and type 2 diabetes. As a result, the diagnosis is very frightening for her and she lacks confidence in her ability to manage her disease. Using empathic responding as well as providing relevant information, how would you address these concerns with Jane?

Case Study 3

The following case illustrates the various interviewing techniques described in Chapter 8.

Patricia Evans is a community pharmacist. A woman she has never seen before approaches the prescription counter with a prescription for an albuterol inhaler for a pediatric patient, Johnny Moore. Analyze the following communication between Patricia and the patient's mother, Ms. Moore.

PATRICIA: Hello. I'm Patricia Evans, the pharmacist here.

MS. MOORE: Hi. I'm Cindy Moore. The prescription is for my son, Johnny.

PATRICIA: Is this the first time you have been to our pharmacy?

MS. MOORE: Yes.

PATRICIA: With people who are coming to our pharmacy for the first time, we like to find out about medications they are currently taking so we can prevent any problems occurring with new medications. If you have about 10 minutes, I'd like to talk with you about the medications Johnny takes. While we're talking, the technician will begin filling your prescription.

MS. MOORE: OK.

PATRICIA: First, how old is Johnny?

Ms. Moore: He's 5 years old.

Patricia: What medical problems does Johnny have?

Ms. Moore: He has asthma. It's really awful. I get so scared when he has an asthma attack.

Patricia: I'm sure with this new medication, we'll be able to prevent those attacks.

Ms. Moore: Yeah. I've heard that before. "Things will get better." Well, things *aren't* getting better.

Patricia: I'm sure your doctor is doing all he can.

Ms. Moore: I'm *sure* he is.

Patricia: What other prescription medications is Johnny currently taking?

Ms. Moore: He is taking Zyrtec syrup for allergies.

Patricia: Do you give the Zytec as prescribed?

Ms. Moore: Of course I do!

Patricia: How well does Johnny take his medicine?

Ms. Moore: He doesn't like to take it. He spits it out. It tastes awful.

Patricia: You're going to have to get him to take it better than that. Otherwise, you can't be sure he's getting the full dose.

Ms. Moore: I bet *you* don't have kids.

Patricia: What other medication does Johnny take?

Ms. Moore: None.

Patricia: Is Johnny allergic to any medication?

Ms. Moore: Yes. He had a reaction to penicillin when he was a baby.

Patricia: What happened when he had the reaction?

Ms. Moore: He got a rash and ran a fever.

Patricia: Any other allergies to medications?

Ms. Moore: No.

Patricia: Let me see if I have everything you've told me—Johnny is taking Zyrtec to treat allergies but does not like to take it. He is allergic to penicillin. Is there anything else you can think of—other medications he takes or problems he has had with medications.

Ms. Moore: No.

Patricia: Now let's discuss the new medication that you will be giving Johnny. . .

Once again, analyze the above communication in terms of positive and negative aspects of Patricia's communication. Examine each of Patricia's responses and Ms. Moore's reaction to her questions. How could questions have been rephrased to be more effective? What questions should have been asked but were not? What could Patricia have said to show more understanding and empathy? What possible drug-related problems were uncovered during the interview? What interventions might Patricia initiate to help resolve these drug-related problems?

Case Study 4

The following case illustrates the technique of asking effective probing questions.

Eleanor Norton is an 80-year-old woman who comes into Paul Singer's pharmacy and presents complaints of insomnia and mild depression. A look at Eleanor's computer profile reveals prescriptions for Premarin (conjugated estrogens), 0.625 mg 1 QD and Provera (medroxyprogesterone), 2.5 mg 1 QD first filled approximately 1.5 years ago. In addition, she has refill records for Desyril (trazodone) 50 mg 1 QHS and Xanax 0.25 mg 1 TID initiated approximately 1 year ago. Refill records are consistent and do not indicate either late or early refills. Complete demographic and allergy information are on the profile, as are notes that indicate the patient does not smoke and does not consume either caffeine or alcohol.

What further information would you want from Ms. Norton to assess her complaints of insomnia and depression? Phrase the exact questions you would ask her to try to obtain this information.

Now analyze the following exchange between Paul and Ms. Norton in which he attempts to assess her complaints.

PAUL: Ms. Norton, I am concerned about your reports of problems sleeping and feelings of depression. I'd like to take about 10 minutes to talk with you about these problems and about the medications you take. This will help me determine things we might do to resolve these problems. Do you have the time now to talk with me?

MS. NORTON: Yes, I do.

PAUL: Good. Let's sit over here where we have more privacy. . . . Now, first tell me when you started experiencing the problems sleeping.

MS. NORTON: About a year ago. I had problems sleeping and felt moody and tired all the time. This is just not like me. I've always been upbeat and very active. Never had a bit of trouble sleeping.

PAUL: Was there anything that happened at that time that might have caused the problem?

Ms. NORTON: Nothing. I've been widowed for 20 years and have gotten used to living alone. My children live nearby and visit nearly every day. Nothing was any different.

PAUL: It must have been frustrating to suddenly feel depressed for no reason you could identify.

Ms. NORTON: It was. I'm not one to sit around and feel sorry for myself all the time.

PAUL: What did you do about the problem at that time?

Ms. NORTON: I told my doctor and he started giving me the trazodone and Xanax to try to get me over it.

PAUL: And how did that work?

Ms. NORTON: I think it did help at first. For several months I seemed to feel better. But then the sleep problems started in again. I am very faithful about taking my medicines but they still didn't seem to do the trick. I told my doctor about it but he didn't change my medicines. I read in *Consumer Reports* about the dangers of Xanax in older people, but he seemed to think I should stick with it a while longer.

PAUL: How do you take the trazodone.

Ms. NORTON: I take it every night at bedtime. Never miss.

PAUL: And the Xanax?

Ms. NORTON: Every 8 hours. I set an alarm so I remember them.

PAUL: Have you had any problems with the use of either of these medicines?

Ms. NORTON: Like side effects? Nothing really. The only problem is they don't seem to work.

PAUL: That must be discouraging.

Ms. NORTON: It is. And I'm on a very tight budget. I can't afford to buy medications that aren't doing me any good.

PAUL: Let's talk more about the symptoms you currently have. Tell me about the problem sleeping.

Ms. NORTON: I have trouble getting to sleep every night but that isn't as bad as waking up at 2:00 and not getting back to sleep until 6:00 and waking up again at 8. This happens almost every night and has been going on for months. I'm tired all day. I used to garden and belonged to clubs and now I don't want to do anything. I don't even invite friends over for lunch like I used to. I'm just too depressed.

Paul: It sounds like the problems sleeping and the depression have changed your life in profound ways.

Ms. Norton: I hate feeling this way. I'm lonely but I know it's because I don't see my friends as much as I used to. I keep hoping the medicines will start working or the doctor will give me something new to take.

Paul: I'll work closely with your doctor to see if we can suggest better treatment for your problems.

Ms. Norton: I'd sure appreciate that.

Paul: Now I'd like to find out about other medications you might take. What other prescription medications do you take?

Ms. Norton: I take Premarin and Provera, one tablet every morning. My doctor prescribed it to prevent osteoporosis.

Paul: When did you first begin taking these medications?

Ms. Norton: Over a year ago. I never bothered to go to a doctor much and didn't start taking hormones when I was younger like most women do. I didn't need them. I still don't seem to have problems—haven't had any broken bones or other problems which, according to what I have read, go along with osteoporosis.

Paul: Do taking the hormones present any problems for you.

Ms. Norton: Not really. I have read that they can cause depression, but when I asked my doctor about it, he told me they were not the cause of my problems.

Paul: I see. Do you take any other prescription medications?

Ms. Norton: No. Nothing.

Paul: Now I'd like to discuss medications you take that you can get without a prescription, in a drug store or grocery store.

Ms. Norton: I don't like to take anything. I'll take Tylenol (acetominophen) if I have a headache, but it has to be pretty bad. I can't remember the last time I've taken anything like that.

Paul: OK. Let me just summarize and you can jump in if I have anything wrong or missed something. You take Premarin and Provera which you started over a year ago. Approximately 1 year ago you started experiencing problems with insomnia and depression. Your doctor prescribed trazodone and Xanax, which seemed to help for several months but then the problems returned. You take no other prescriptions and rarely use nonprescription medications. . . Is there anything else you can think of regarding your use of medications?

Ms. Norton: No. That's all I can think of.

Paul: Thank you. This information helps me keep track of how you are responding to your treatment. Often, we can't know if a medicine is the best one for you unless we try it and see how it works. I will be communicating with your doctor as soon as I can about your sleep problems and depression and together we'll try to come up with something that is effective in overcoming these problems. I don't want to keep you waiting longer today. I'll call you within the week to discuss our recommendation with you. Will that be OK. with you?

Ms. Norton: I'd really appreciate that. Sometimes I'm so flustered when I see my doctor that I don't remember to tell him everything.

Paul: And if you think of anything when you get home, or if you have any concerns about your treatment, please call me. I'll give you my card with my phone number on it . . . Do you have anything you'd like to discuss right now?

Ms. Norton: No. The sleep problem is the main thing I want resolved and we've discussed that pretty thoroughly. I see my doctor in 2 weeks, so I hope he can do something then to help me.

Now critique Paul's interview depicted above. What were the strengths and weaknesses of his communication skills? What further information do you think he should have obtained from Ms. Norton? How empathic did he seem?

After Paul concluded his interview with Ms. Norton he decided to intervene with the prescribing physician. Since the problems Ms. Norton reported had been ongoing and did not present an emergency situation, Paul decided he could best communicate with the physician in the consult letter on the next page, which he faxed to the physician's office, rather than consulting with the physician over the phone.

Now critique Paul's letter asking the following questions. What was the tone that Paul was trying to set with the physician? What are the positive aspects of the way Paul approached the communication? What changes would you have made to improve the effectiveness of the written communication?

An effective consultation letter should contain the following attributes:

1. The correspondence should be typed on pharmacy letterhead should be personalized addressing a specific patient and physician rather than having the feel of a "form letter."

2. It should contain the following information:
   a. Patient name
   b. Date of communication with patient or date of review of patient medication use
   c. Concerns expressed by the patient or uncovered in drug use review

    d. Identification of any verified or potential drug-related problem (this could include misuse of the medication by the patient, presence of a possible medical problem not currently being treated, or problems related to current medication therapy)

    e. Clarification of the optimal therapeutic outcome

    f. Description of appropriate alternative approaches to resolving drug-related problem(s)

    g. Recommendations as to the preferred alternative and specific recommendations for implementation (e.g., dosing recommendations for selected drugs) which are tailored to the patient's needs

    h. Suggestions for an appropriate monitoring plan, along with specific actions you will undertake to assist in monitoring patient response

3. Any recommendations should be supported with citations from current, accepted literature sources.

4. The letter should encourage future two-way dialogue with the physician.

5. The tone must emphasize helping the patient rather than promoting the pharmacist.

Case Study 5

Since the incidence of HIV infection is rising worldwide, particularly in heterosexual women, adolescents, and intravenous. drug users, pharmacists, like any other health professional, have a responsibility to be well educated regarding this disease. Respond to the following scenario:

This situation takes place in the small rural town that has a county hospital, about 10 physicians, and two pharmacies (one chain and one independent pharmacy). The case involves David Johnson, a 6-year-old child who tested positive for HIV 2 years ago and 6 months ago showed slight symptoms of Pneumocystis carinii pneumonia. *Since that time he has been given Bactrim suspension (sulfamethoxasole) prophylaxically (1 teaspoonful daily). The Johnsons recently moved to town.*

Mrs. Johnson and David enter Fred Schneider's pharmacy for the first time to obtain a new supply of Bactrim and also some Tylenol with Codeine elixir. Fred was expecting David since he heard that a young kid with AIDS and his mother had moved into town. Mrs. Johnson approached the prescription counter and greeted Fred with a warm smile. Fred kind of grunted "good morning" as he took the prescriptions. The following conversation transpired:

August 8, 2002

Russell N. Sellers, M.D.
1616 N. 50 St
Cooperstown, NY

Dear Dr. Sellers:

Yesterday I spoke with one of your patients, Eleanor Norton, who conveyed to me her concerns about problems with insomnia and depression. She reported that the trazodone and Xanax you prescribed for her condition seemed to work for several months, but then the symptoms returned. The symptoms have led her to severely restrict her activities and contacts with friends, which she reports has had a negative effect on her quality of life. I would like to work with you to devise an alternative treatment for Ms. Norton that might relieve the symptoms she reports. I can assist you in closely monitoring her response to treatment to see if changes we make resolve the problem.

I believe there are three alternative avenues we might explore to resolve the patient's problems. The focus might be on altering the hormone replacement therapy, on choosing an alternate antidepressant such as fluoxetine, or on altering the benzodiazepine therapy. The onset of depressive symptoms shortly after initiation of hormone replacement therapy suggests the possibility that the hormone therapy is causing the depression. I, therefore, think this should be our first line of attack. I am enclosing a recent article that suggests that hormone replacement therapy may not be necessary in women over 75 with no history of bone fractures or other indications of severe osteoporosis. The authors note that most of the loss of bone density occurs prior to age 75. They also review the evidence that a side effect for many patients is depression. The recommendation of these authors is use of calcium and Vitamin D supplements only. While there is certainly variation in medical practice on this issue, I think the decreased quality of life of Ms. Norton due to the depression, which could be tied to the hormone therapy, makes an alternative treatment worth considering. You may feel more confident in making this decision if a bone density evaluation of Ms. Norton was first conducted. My only concern here would be with the cost of the procedure given the limited income Ms. Norton reports.

If you decide to discontinue hormone replacement therapy, I plan to call Ms. Norton every two weeks to assess her response to the alteration and will update you on her progress. If she responds well, we could then discuss gradually reducing and eventually eliminating the trazodone and Xanax. If response is not as we would hope, we could then discuss an alternative approach to address the problem. Ms. Norton informed me that she has an appointment to see you in 2 weeks. Please keep me informed of any changes that you make in her therapy so that I may be of as much assistance as possible.

I hope to be able to work with you in helping Ms. Norton. I welcome the opportunity to discuss alternative approaches to resolving Ms. Norton's depression. Please call me at your earliest convenience.

Sincerely,

Paul T. Singer

Paul T. Singer, Pharm.D.

FRED: What are these for?

MRS. JOHNSON: Something for his lungs. One of them helps with the pain.

FRED: Well, these medications may help for awhile, but they are not going to cure him.

Fred retreated behind the prescription counter and gave the prescriptions to his assistant so that the labels could be typed while he prepared the drugs.

ASSISTANT: Mrs. Johnson, who's the doctor anyway? I can't read his handwriting.

MRS. JOHNSON: That would be Dr. Dennis. He was seeing David in the town where we used to live.

FRED (TO THE ASSISTANT): Can't fill these, they might be forgeries. They should come from a local doctor, but I don't know who will treat an AIDS patient, especially when the mother is probably a drug addict.

FRED: Mrs. Johnson, I'm sorry you'll have to get these written by a local physician. I could recommend Dr. Wright; he sees most of the Medicaid patients here in town. His office is next to the county hospital.

MRS. JOHNSON: I thought I could get these filled anywhere. I'd rather not run around all over town with David.

FRED: Sorry, rules are rules. We close tonight at 9:00 PM sharp. Bye.
Mrs. Johnson and David exit the pharmacy.

What stereotypes did Fred have of the patient?
How did these stereotypes influence his behavior?
If you were Fred's supervisor, what would you say to him regarding this interaction?

Obviously, Fred's unprofessional behavior is unacceptable and if allowed to continue, could destroy the ability of anyone in the pharmacy to establish helpful relationships with Mrs. Johnson.

Case Study 6

A women enters the pharmacy to discuss the following situation:

> *"I recently found a prescription for penicillin for my boyfriend from the county's STD (sexually transmitted diseases) clinic. This prescription was filled at this pharmacy 3 days ago and I want to know what it is used for. What's going on here?"*

What would you say to this patient?
What important communication issues are involved?
What is your role in this situation?

Case Study 7

A husband comes into your pharmacy to discuss a problem his wife has been having lately.

> *"My wife has been taking a tranquilizer, diazepam I believe, for about 4 months after she pinched a nerve in the back of her neck at work. She has been acting strangely lately and I am afraid she is becoming addicted to this drug. She is also drinking more than she used to. She seems to be very moody (anxious one moment and quiet the next). I went through her things and found several prescription bottles from different physicians and from other pharmacies. What should I do? Is there any hope?"*

What would you say to this husband?
How would you phrase your questions?
What is your role in this interaction?
Would you call anyone else about this? If so, who?

Case Study 8

Bob Holiday is a 40-year-old male who suffers from seasonal allergies. His allergies have become worse since he moved to a state well known for its bothersome plant life. Typically, his eyes become watery and red, his nose runs, and he has a mild headache. Today he reports that these symptoms appeared along with a sore throat and a more severe headache. He felt he had a strep throat and so he sought the services of a physician. The physician assured him the symptoms were his allergies "kicking up" and that the sore throat and headache were due to sinus drainage. The physician gave Bob the following prescription:

Bob Holiday
Rx: Allegra D Tab
#60
Sig: i am, i pm,
J. Smith MD

What should you verify before and after filling this prescription?
What would you say to keep the counseling encounter to less than a minute and still fulfill your counseling obligations?

By using a few simple open-ended questions, you could verify that the medication is being taken for seasonal allergies, even though Bob's physical appearance probably suggests it. Also verification that these symptoms are not the side effects of any other OTC or Rx medication is needed. Finally, through open-ended questions you should verify that the patient understands the directions for use and any anticipated side effects such as drowsiness.

Case Study 9

You are a pharmacist working in community pharmacy. Mrs. Elliott enters the prescription area to pick up a medication. Mrs. Elliott is a relatively new patient to your pharmacy and has been taking medication for high blood pressure for about 4 years. You hand her the prescription and say, "I notice that it has been a while since you last got this medication refilled."

Answer the following questions regarding this situation:

1. In communicating with Mrs. Elliott, which aspect of communication contributes the most in the transmission of your message to her?
    a. Level of empathy
    b. Tone of voice
    c. Nonverbal aspects
    d. Amount of privacy
    e. b and c

2. Mrs. Elliott seems to be reluctant to answer your direct questions about her compliance with her high blood pressure medication. What type of questions should you ask to draw her out?
    a. Open-ended
    b. Closed-ended
    c. Leading
    d. None of the above

3. Mrs. Elliott's reluctance to speak with you may be due to her perception of you as a pharmacist. Which of the following could result in distortions in interpersonal perception?

   a. Conflicting values

   b. Stereotyping

   c. Personal concerns

   d. All of the above

   e. None of the above

4. Mrs. Elliott states, "I'm tired of taking this medication. Sometimes I don't take them like I should." You respond by saying, "How long have you been taking this medication, Mrs. Elliott? Are they causing you any particular side effects?" Your response is an example of what type of response?

   a. Advising

   b. Quizzing

   c. Analyzing

   d. Evaluating

   e. Focusing

5. You go on to say, "Now, Mrs. Elliott, you shouldn't worry too much about that. It happens to a lot of people. Everything will work out if you take your medications correctly." This is an example of what type of response?

   a. Advising

   b. Reassuring

   c. Warning

   d. Judging

   e. Understanding

Answers to questions: 1, e. 2, a. 3, d. 4, b. 5, b.

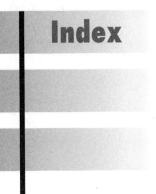

Index

In this index, page numbers in *italics* designate figures; page numbers followed by the letter "t" designate boxes or tables. *See also* cross references designate related topics of more detailed subentries.